THE POWER OF
puberty & periods

THE KNOWLEDGE

THE POWER OF
puberty & periods

BY DR NIGHAT ARIF

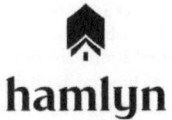

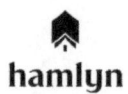
hamlyn

First published as *The Power of Puberty & Periods*
in Great Britain in 2025 by Hamlyn,
an imprint of
Octopus Publishing Group Ltd
Carmelite House
50 Victoria Embankment
London EC4Y 0DZ
www.octopusbooks.co.uk

An Hachette UK Company
www.hachette.co.uk

The authorized representative in the EEA is Hachette Ireland,
8 Castlecourt Centre, Dublin 15, D15 XTP3, Ireland (email: info@hbgi.ie)

This material was previously published as *The Knowledge:
Your guide to female health from menstruation to the menopause* by Aster in 2023

Text copyright © Dr Nighat Arif 2025

All rights reserved. No part of this work may be reproduced or utilized in any form or by any means, electronic or mechanical, including photocopying, recording or by any information storage and retrieval system, without the prior written permission of the publisher.

Dr Nighat Arif has asserted their right under the Copyright,
Designs and Patents Act 1988 to be identified as the author of this work.

ISBN 978-0-60063-970-1
eISBN 978-0-60063-971-8

A CIP catalogue record for this book is available from the British Library.

Typeset in 10.5/15pt Sabon LT Pro by Six Red Marbles UK, Thetford, Norfolk

Printed and bound in Great Britain.

1 3 5 7 9 10 8 6 4 2

This FSC® label means that materials used for the product have
been responsibly sourced.

Disclaimer: Before making any changes in your health regime, or starting any medical treatment, always consult your own doctor for advice relevant to your individual circumstances.

Staff Credits:
Publisher: Kate Fox
Senior Editor: Pauline Bache
Art Director: Jaz Bahra
Words Contributor: Joanne Lake
Illustrator: Liliana Rasmussen
Picture Research: Giulia Hetherington and Jennifer Veall
Copy Editor: Joanne Smith
Production Manager: Caroline Alberti

CONTENTS

Your guide to female health	1
Female anatomy & self examinations	9
Fair healthcare access for all	37

Puberty & Periods

Introduction	59
Physical changes during puberty	63
Periods	65
Period inequality	89
Let's talk about periods	91
Cultural attitudes towards menstruation	97
Health & comfort issues during your monthly cycle	103
Violence against women & girls	117
Caring for your vulva & vagina	119
Infections of the genitals & urinary tract	125
Sexual health & contraception	131
Unplanned pregnancy	157
Sexually transmitted diseases	161
Considerations for trans individuals	167
Dr Nighat's takeaways	173

Sharing the knowledge	174
Glossary of women's health	176
Resources	188
Index	192
Acknowledgements	196
About the author	201

YOUR GUIDE TO FEMALE HEALTH

Back in the spring of 2019, I was working at a practice in rural Buckinghamshire as a GP with a special interest in women's health. That area of medicine had always fascinated me, from menstruation through to menopause, and helping people to access the right care and treatment had become my vocation and my passion.

Alongside my GP duties, I began to create social media posts to raise awareness of various topics: the importance of cervical screening, for instance, or the benefits of HRT. I wanted to use my experience as a clinician to empower women with knowledge, to encourage them to get to know their bodies and to dispel the myths that were often perpetuated within the area of women's health. To communicate these important messages in the most effective manner possible, I took great care to use clear language, factual terminology and evidence-based data. Furthermore, as someone with Pakistani heritage, I was keen to reach out to a South Asian audience, so I produced content in Urdu and Punjabi as well as English.

My tweets, TikTok and Instagram posts began to gather momentum and soon caught the attention of the BBC. In May 2019, they invited me onto the show to discuss the common symptoms of menopause and my efforts to raise awareness in the ethnic minority community. This appearance by a 30-something, hijab-wearing Muslim woman caused quite a stir, not just because I was talking openly about night sweats and vaginal dryness – considered taboo subjects by many – on a flagship TV programme, but also because GPs who looked like me were rarely seen on TV. The positive feedback I received as a consequence – especially from women of colour – completely blew me away.

More TV appearances followed (including on ITV) and my social media hits skyrocketed. I received thousands of responses from people across the globe who had watched one of my videos, recognized their own symptoms and – armed with new-found information – had checked in with a healthcare professional. As a GP this was music to my ears, of course, but it also highlighted a huge demand for clear, factual and accessible advice. And that, in a nutshell, is what prompted me to grab my laptop and write *The Knowledge*.

I want to share my expertise. I want to start a conversation. I want you to understand your body, to identify any changes and to realize when – and how – to seek help. Ultimately, I want you to look after yourself in the best way possible so you can lead a long, happy and healthy life. It is so important to me that women of all ages are able to advocate for themselves and get the best healthcare possible. So this series of books will cover women through every stage of life, from Puberty, to their Fertile Years, into Midlife and beyond. However, there are some elements of female health that truly do transcend the ages – I'm thinking of the need to understand your body, know your rights, and be aware of lifelong health checks.

So, this essential information is included at the front of all books in this series – to provide a comprehensive guide to female health at every stage of life.

I firmly believe that everyone assigned female at birth, regardless of age, should learn about the three distinct phases and the changes they embrace. Indeed, during the writing process I found it helpful to view things from the perspective of my 14-year-old self. I was raised in a traditional, religious Muslim household where women's health matters were hardly discussed, so I had to use other means to learn about things like menstruation and contraception. The teenage 'me' would have undoubtedly appreciated a book like this, as it would have given me a deeper understanding of myself . . . and a deeper understanding of my mother and grandmother!

And while I want to help women and girls of all ages, I'm just as keen to help their loved ones, too – that's mums, dads, siblings, grandparents and other relatives or caregivers. I particularly want to reach out to fathers, perhaps those who are single, separated or widowed – or in same-sex relationships – who may not have female partners to consult. It's so important that you feel comfortable talking to your daughters about period products, or family planning, and can do so openly and honestly.

Removing the shame and stigma from women's health is an ongoing mission of mine and forms a central theme of these books. The embarrassment factor can prove to be fatal, quite literally, if it prevents someone from getting the right care at the right time. Gynaecological cancers claim thousands of lives each year but, by performing self examinations of your breast tissue, vulva and vagina – and having regular smear tests – any changes or anomalies may be spotted early enough for you to obtain successful treatment. We also need to encourage our children and young people to familiarize themselves with their genitals without feeling ashamed. By normalizing these matters – girls checking their vulvas, boys checking their penises – good habits will be formed and infection and disease may be averted. So much of my work as a GP involves this kind of preventative care; it genuinely does save lives.

This series also offers help and advice for individuals who don't fit the mould of what society – and the healthcare system – still deem as 'normal' (although I always question this concept, because in medicine there's no such thing as a 'normal' period, for example, or a 'normal' menopause). I'm very proud of the fact that this book includes guidance for trans people and those with disabilities. These individuals have exactly the same rights to sexual and reproductive healthcare as any other patient, and should receive treatment without discrimination or prejudice. This content may also be useful to fellow clinicians, who should be ensuring their surgeries and consultations are as inclusive and as accessible as possible.

I apply a similar principle to people struggling with infertility or baby loss, whose circumstances should never be overlooked or underplayed. Successful conception, pregnancy and childbirth is still very much part of the common narrative, meaning that those who encounter problems often feel excluded from the conversation. Many women of colour can feel side-lined, too; institutional racism, combined with systemic misogyny, continues to prevail in the healthcare sector and I still hear appalling stories from women of colour whose symptoms are dismissed and whose pain is invalidated. I'm determined to combat this, and will continue to call for allies to fight our corner and for ambassadors to connect with communities.

And let me be clear: should anyone query why inclusivity, diversity and ally-ship is so important to me, and why it forms such an intrinsic part of my ethos (and this book), I'll always flip it around to ask, 'Well, why shouldn't it be important? And why should the question even need to be asked in the first place?' As far as I'm concerned, the basic principles of medicine are universal. Gold-standard healthcare should be available to all. No one should face bias or exclusion; on the contrary, they should all have a place at the table.

As a member of an ethnic group, and an employee of the UK's National Health Service (NHS), the issue of representation really matters to me. It's a known fact that most promotional healthcare material – leaflets, posters, diagrams and illustrations – does not always feature people of colour. This, quite understandably, can send the wrong signals to people who may already feel excluded from mainstream medicine, and who are therefore less likely to engage with clinicians. I'm doing my utmost to challenge and change this, and am immensely proud of the illustrations that have been specially created for this book. I only wish they'd existed when I was younger; back then, public health messaging was distinctly white, Western and middle class.

I'm also keen to break down the cultural barriers that prevent women of colour from accessing the care they need. Many of their health issues, including menstruation and menopause, are kept 'under the veil' (not spoken about, in other words), which can have a severe impact on their wellbeing. To these people – and to anybody else who's feeling alone and isolated – I truly hope I can help you to find your voice and start that conversation.

But along with being heard, you also need to feel seen. And as someone who eats, sleeps and breathes clinical medicine, I want all women to know that I see them, whether suffering with endometriosis, living with perimenopause, coping with infertility, struggling with gender identity, or simply wanting to be sure that their periods are normal. This book, I hope, will empower you to get the healthcare you deserve and, not only that, will encourage you to spread the word and tell your story. Your knowledge is a gift, to be shared freely with others. I hope this book plays a role in providing a pillar of support on that journey. You may not find every single answer within these pages – medicine is rarely one-size-fits-all, and no two people experience the same symptoms – but if you spot a nugget of advice that prompts you to pick up the phone to your doctor, or encourages you to perform your first self examination, then this labour of love will have served its purpose.

Finally, each one of us carries a candle of knowledge. Kindled by wisdom and experience, it brings light, warmth and energy. But we shouldn't keep the candle to ourselves. We should use it to light somebody else's. That way, the flame continues to burn brightly.

With love,

Dr Nighat Arif

Dear body, thank you for harbouring me, making me beautiful, nourishing me, making me capable of remarkable things. I promise to love and respect you.

FEMALE ANATOMY & SELF EXAMINATIONS

Awareness of your own body is key to good health, so it's vital that you educate yourself about your basic anatomy, both internal and external. In every book in this series, I have included the following pages with diagrams of the internal female reproductive system and breasts, as well as a diagram of the external vulva and pubic area. These should really help as a reference point for many sections of the book that follow.

While much of your internal anatomy won't be visible to you, it is still vital that you have a keen awareness of how areas of your body look and feel – because every body is different, only you can know your own body best. If I had my own way, every woman or person assigned female at birth (AFAB) would examine their breast tissue and genitals on a regular basis from the age of 13. Ideally, by the time you are 18, you should complete all self examinations once a month, in between periods. The more we learn about the way we look, and the way things feel, the more likely we'll be to notice changes and spot anomalies. Flagging up any concerns to your doctor may help them recognize certain symptoms and make early (sometimes life-saving) diagnoses. Pages 19–23 and 31–5 will show you how to undertake these self examinations in detail.

The female reproductive system

The female reproductive system includes everything involved in creating and carrying a baby, but it is so important to have an awareness of your system at every stage of your life, even if you never intend to have a pregnancy. The system begins at the vulva, the external element that you can see in your self examination (see pages 14–15), then moves into the vagina and then the cervix, which is the opening to the uterus. The uterus is lined with the endometrium and is where, if you are pregnant, the foetus will grow and be supported throughout your pregnancy. If you are not pregnant, then your menstrual cycle runs through a process of thickening the endometrium and then shedding the lining with your period. The ovaries are where an egg (ovum) matures each month, which is then released into the fallopian tube to travel along towards the uterus.

FEMALE ANATOMY & SELF EXAMINATIONS

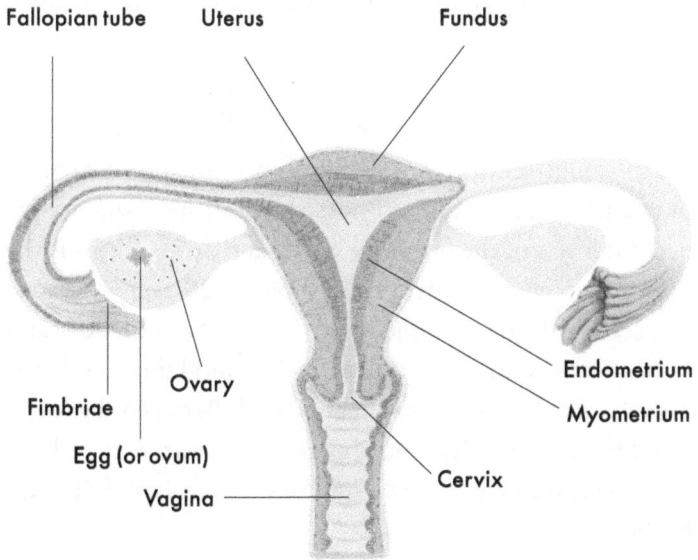

The female reproductive system (side view)

People are frequently surprised by how close the reproductive system is to the lower part of the digestive system, but they are all snugly clustered together within the pelvis. This is particularly important to note during times when your natural levels of the hormone oestrogen drop, as this is the reason why vaginal atrophy (see page 129 and Glossary) can cause infections in the urinary tract. Your bladder and urethra sit just in front of your uterus and labia, while the bowel, rectum and anus sit just behind. Between the lower opening of the vulva and the anus is an area called the perineum, which can easily split or become sore if the skin becomes dry.

FEMALE ANATOMY & SELF EXAMINATIONS

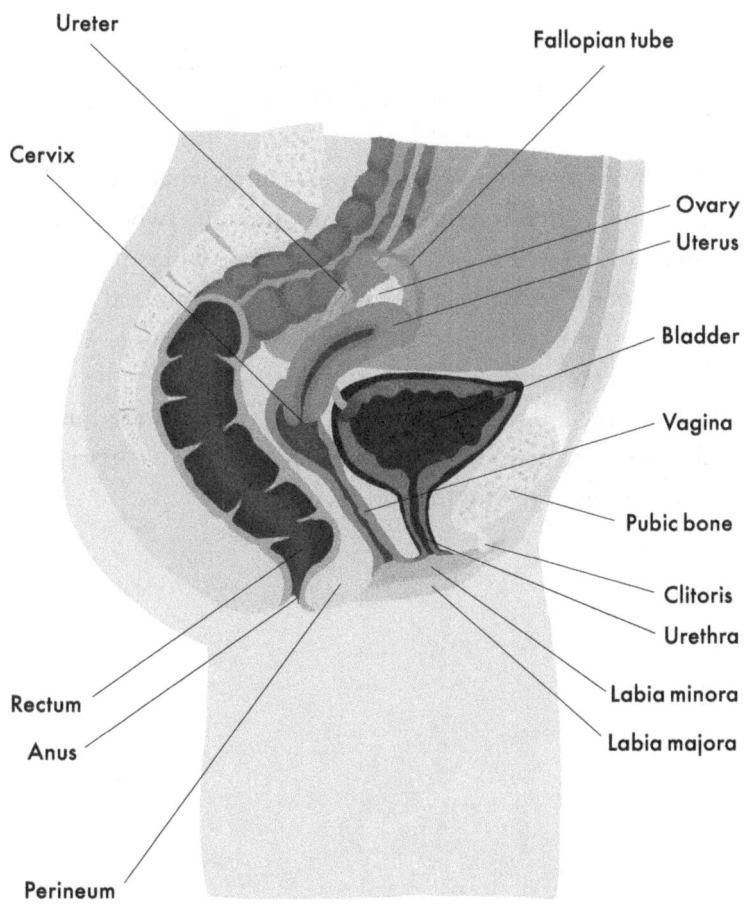

The vulva & pubic area

The vulva is the external part of your genitals while the pubic area is that between your legs, above your vulva, where your pubic hair grows. Looking into the vulva you will see that it's formed of the outer labia and inner labia. The clitoral hood sits at the top of the inner labia and covers the clitoris, while the urethral opening (where you urinate from) is just below. The entrance to the vagina sits at the bottom of the inner labia, then the perineum is the area of skin that sits between the openings of the vagina and the anus.

FEMALE ANATOMY & SELF EXAMINATIONS

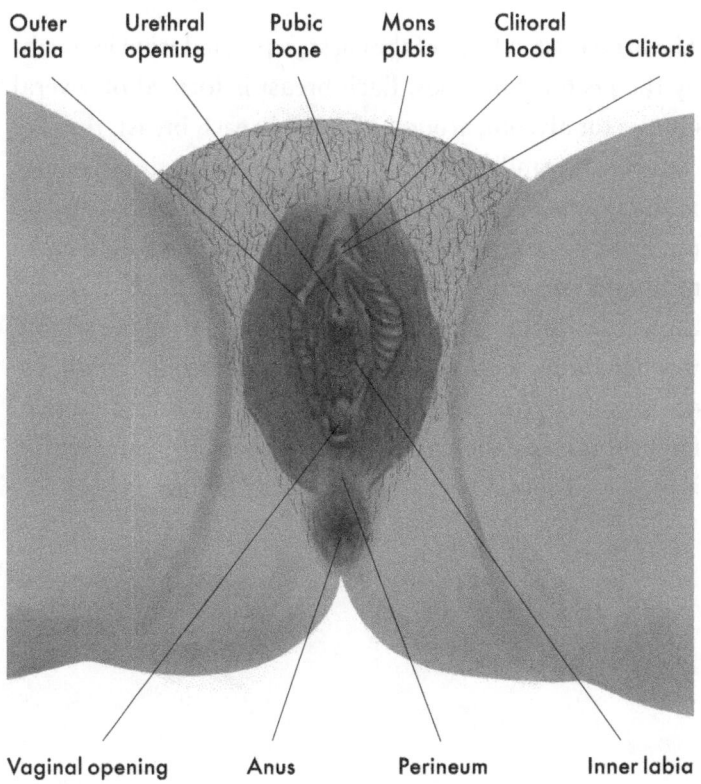

The breast

The breasts sit in front of the chest, separated from your ribs by the pectoral muscles. Each breast is formed of several lobules (or alveoli), around 15 to 20 in each breast, that are connected via milk ducts and milk reservoirs to tiny openings in the nipple. The hormonal changes associated with late pregnancy and childbirth will stimulate the alveoli to make milk and the action of a baby suckling at the breast will cause a 'let down', when the milk is released from the alveoli, through the milk ducts and reservoirs out through the nipple openings. The first milk that comes from the breast is a rich, fatty substance called colostrum and then the 'mature' milk is produced about two days after a baby is born.

FEMALE ANATOMY & SELF EXAMINATIONS

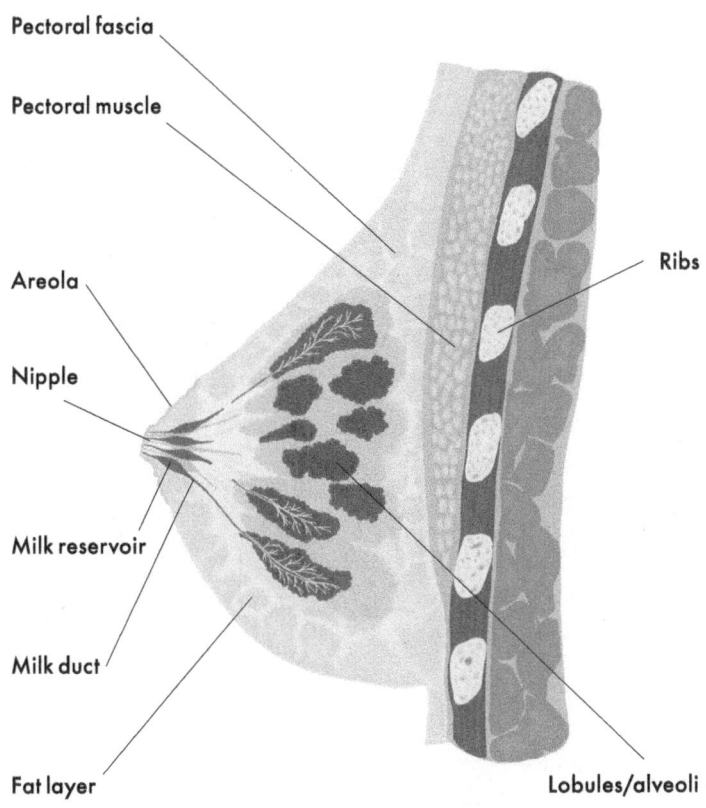

SELF EXAMINATION: BREASTS

Breast cancer is very common and, in the UK, about one in seven women will be diagnosed with it in their lifetime. Early detection significantly improves the chance of successful treatment and recovery, which is why it is so important to examine your breast tissue on a regular basis. Thanks to the increased raising of awareness throughout the NHS – and the fabulous work of charities like Breast Cancer Now – more women are examining their breast tissue than ever before. A thorough self examination should take about ten minutes and might just save your life.

Examining your breasts

I advise my patients to do breast examinations on a monthly basis: on roughly the same date each month, or two weeks before or after your period if you're menstruating (as fluctuations in oestrogen around your period are likely to cause breast pain and swelling that might mean missing any lumps).

Perform your breast exam wherever it feels comfortable (preferably somewhere nice and quiet, where you won't be disturbed) – perhaps on your bed, or in the bath or shower. I often tell my patients to do it at a particular time of day, which might help to jog their memory and make it a routine, perhaps in front of their bedroom mirror as they're getting dressed for work on a Monday morning. I know some women who ask their partners to have a good feel of their breast tissue – you'd be surprised how many lumps are found by loved ones – and you can always return the favour by assisting with their personal examinations. It's important to point out that those assigned male at birth can get breast cancer too, so it's a good idea for them to check their pecs regularly.

Breast implants can make a self examination more difficult but it is still important. You should be able to gently shift the position of the implant and you can then palpate around the implant to feel the breast tissue around it.

What to look out for during a breast self examination
- A new lump in the breast or armpit area, which may or may not cause pain.
- Irritation, redness, darkening or flaking of the skin around the breast and nipple area.
- A swelling or thickening in any part of the breast.
- Skin snagging, puckering or dimpling around the nipple area.
- Nipple discharge or blood if not pregnant or nursing.
- A marked and visible change in breast size (it's common for women to have one breast bigger than the other, but watch out for *recent* changes).
- A dull or sharp pain in any area of the breast.

Try to focus and concentrate as you feel your breasts. Don't be half-hearted or absent-minded! Remind yourself that you're feeling for lumps and bumps in the breast tissue

SELF EXAMINATION: BREASTS

and armpit area, and are looking for any changes in the skin or nipple.

If you *do* notice any irregularities during a self examination, try not to panic or assume the worst. Make a note of these changes, however small, and book an appointment to see your doctor as soon as possible, outlining the reasons to the receptionist when you call.

Do not delay matters or tell yourself that you're worrying unnecessarily. The sooner you get seen by a clinician, the better. And – should anything require further investigation – you'll be promptly referred to a specialist.

How to examine your breasts

Examine your breast tissue monthly, preferably between your periods. Find somewhere you are comfortable, either standing up or lying on your back. Then remove your top and bra. Complete the following steps on both sides.

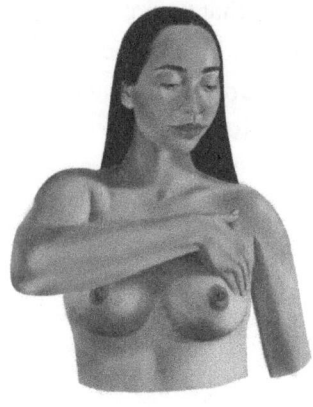 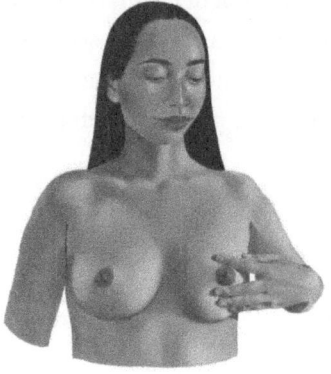

1 With the pads of four fingers, slowly press around the fleshy breast tissue in a circular motion, moving outwards from the nipple to your rib and armpit areas. Apply pressure that's firm, but comfortable. Feel for any changes to the flesh or skin as outlined opposite.

2 Use your fingers to feel underneath and around the nipple, looking for any changes to the flesh or skin.

SELF EXAMINATION: BREASTS

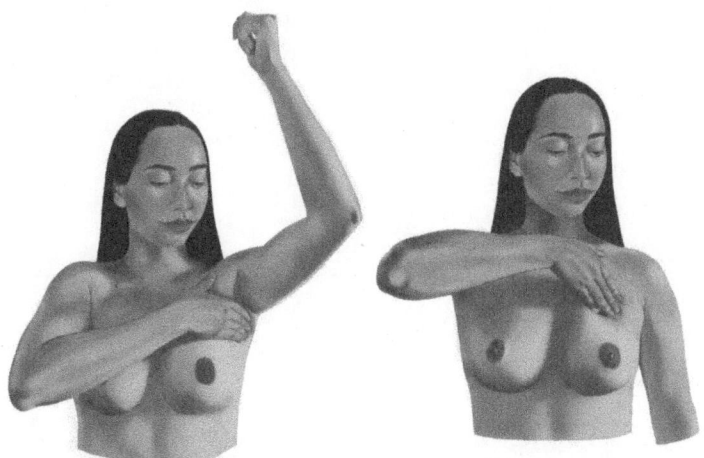

3 Use your fingers to feel underneath the armpit, looking for any changes to the flesh or skin.

4 Walk your fingers up your chest towards your neck, feeling as you go, looking for any changes to the flesh or skin.

WEAR THE CORRECT SIZE BRA!

I see so many women in my surgery with chronic breast pain who are clearly wearing the wrong-sized bra. When I was younger, I never received any guidance about the importance of wearing the right bra. I was none the wiser until the age of 23, when a lovely lady in the lingerie department of a local shop introduced me to the joys (and comfort) of wearing a correctly fitted bra!

The easiest way to find your bra size is to visit the lingerie section of your local department store, or a stand-alone lingerie store. The staff there will be specially trained in measuring busts. Many bra-fitters now determine your size on sight, without a tape measure – a real specialist skill! If, however, you don't feel comfortable visiting a store, or can't find the time to, then you can measure yourself at home, and calculate your bra size from there.

How to measure your bra size

You'll need to take two measurements to determine your bra size: the band measurement and the cup measurement. If possible measure in inches (because that's how bra sizes are calculated), but you can use an online calculator to convert from centimetres if your tape measure doesn't show inches.

To find the band size, measure all around your ribcage just beneath your breasts. (If the measurement is an odd number then scale up or down to the nearest even number.)

This number is your band size. Then measure all around the widest area of your bust, so the tape measure sits firmly but comfortably. Subtracting your band size from this bust measurement will give your cup size, so less than 1 inch (2.5cm) = AA, 1 inch (2.5cm) = A, 2 inches (5cm) = B, 3 inches (7.5cm) = C, 4 inches (10cm) = D, 5 inches (12.7cm) = DD, 6 inches (15.2cm) = E, 7 inches (17.8cm) = F, 8 inches (20.3cm) = FF, 9 inches (22.9cm) = G, 10 inches (25.4cm) = GG, 11 inches (27.9cm) = H. Sizes beyond H are usually available from specialist retailers.

What to look for in a well-fitting bra
- It should be snug when on the loosest hook.
- The shoulder strap should sit comfortably to prevent shoulder pain.
- The cups should be flush with your bust.
- The centre wire or fabric should sit flat against the chest wall; if it pulls away the cup is not deep enough, and if it wobbles the cup is too deep.
- At the sides, the bra wire or fabric should sit under the breast along the ribs; if it sits on the breast tissue, the cup is too small, and if the side wire is too big it will dig into the underarm area.

Cup size = measurement 1 minus measurement 2

How to measure your bra size

Find somewhere you can measure yourself comfortably without being distracted, then either measure over a soft (non-padded) bra – whichever bra you currently find most comfortable to wear – or against your bare breasts.

1 Measure the circumference around the fullest part of your breasts (shown by the solid line in the image on page 29). The tape measure should have a little give in this measurement.

2 Measure the circumference around your ribcage beneath your breasts (shown by the dotted line in the image on page 29). The tape measure should be very snug, but still comfortable for this measurement.

3 Calculate your bra size using the formula on page 26.

WEAR THE CORRECT SIZE BRA!

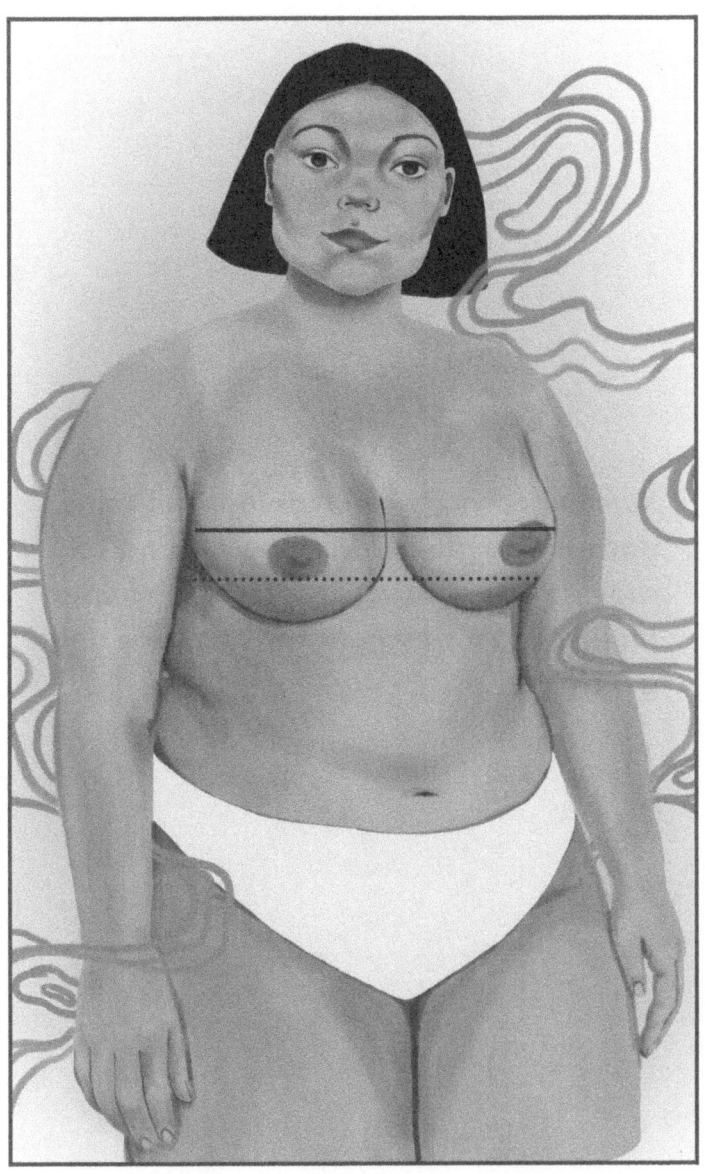

Remember: no two vulvas look the same, each is completely unique. And no one should know your vulva and vagina better than you. So why not grab a mirror and get started?

SELF EXAMINATION: VULVA & PUBIC AREA

Whilst breast self examinations have become commonplace – and have saved countless lives – there is still a huge lack of awareness around genital self examinations. This simply has to change if we are going to reduce the incidence of vaginal and vulval cancers, so it is vital you familiarize yourself with your vulva and pubic area.

Examining your vulva & pubic area

Vulval and vaginal cancers are rare but frequently missed or misdiagnosed. They can occur in women of any age, more often among those who are long-term smokers or who have a family history of melanoma (a type of skin cancer). There are 1,400 new cases of vulval cancer each year in the UK and five every week of vaginal cancer. While they are awful diseases, if picked up early, then the prognoses are encouraging. Self examination is key and, as per usual, this is a euphemism-free zone, so no talk of foo-foos or front bottoms whatsoever!

Not to be confused with the vagina, the vulva is another name for your external genitals, namely the labia majora (outer lips), the labia minora (inner lips) and the clitoris. Speaking as a doctor who has examined thousands of women, I can assure you that no two vulvas look alike.

Becoming familiar with the way your vulva looks and feels is very, very important.

If we're going to raise awareness about vulval examinations, however, we first have to remove the stigma and take away the sexualization of women's bodies in today's society. Examining and touching your vulva for health purposes isn't remotely pornographic – it's a sensible thing to do, not a sexual thing to do – and we need the men in our lives to respect and support us in this regard.

We also need to reach the stage where we can encourage our children to regularly examine their genitals without embarrassment. By normalizing things – girls checking their vulvas every week, boys checking their penises and testicles – good habits will be formed and infections and diseases may be recognized and treated at an early stage.

A vulval examination should ideally take place monthly: on roughly the same date each month, similarly to a breast examination (I often encourage my patients to get into the routine of doing the examinations one after the other). You'll need some privacy – and won't want interruptions, of course – so perhaps choose a locked bathroom or bedroom, preferably with some natural light. Find yourself a small hand-held mirror, and set aside ten minutes or so.

What to look out for during a vulva & pubic region self examination

- Any lumps, bumps, spots or sores that could indicate infection, disease or other conditions.

SELF EXAMINATION: VULVA & PUBIC AREA

- Any changes to the colour or size of different areas from one examination to the next.
- Any bad-smelling discharge (though some discharge is normal, and the amount will depend on what point you are at in your menstrual cycle). If your discharge has a bad smell or is an unusual colour (see pages 121–3) it could indicate an infection.

How to examine your vulva & pubic region

Examine your vulva monthly, preferably between your menstrual periods, if you have them. Before you begin, wash your hands with soap and water, then grab a hand-held mirror and find somewhere with enough space to sit, squat or lie down, on the floor or on a chair, and sufficient light for you to see well, where you won't be interrupted for ten minutes.

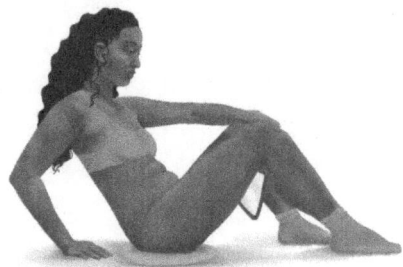

1 Open your legs and check the area where your pubic hair grows. Feel around with your fingers and position your mirror to check for moles, bumps, spots, warts, ulcers, lesions, rashes or white patches. Make a mental note of anything that looks new or feels different. Examine the fleshy area from top to bottom.

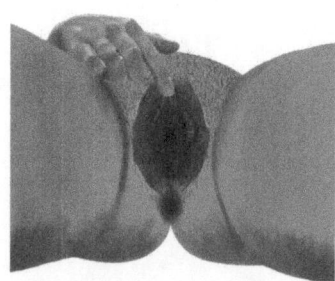

2 Next, find your clitoris – at the top of the vulva, the fold of skin where the inner labia meet – and look for any bumps, growths or discolouration.

SELF EXAMINATION: VULVA & PUBIC AREA

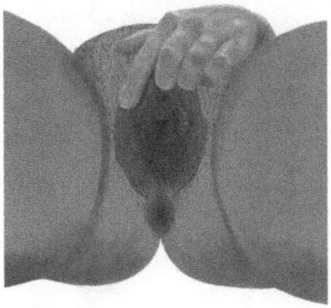

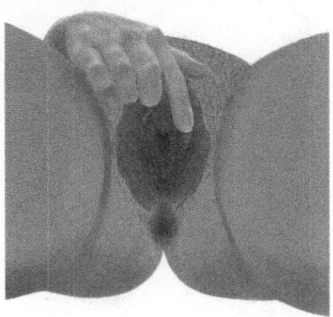

3 Check your labia majora – the outer lips – and, again, feel for any bumps, spots, lesions or rashes.

4 Check your labia minora – the inner lips – and, again, feel for any bumps, spots, lesions or rashes.

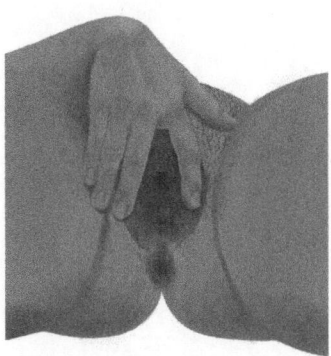

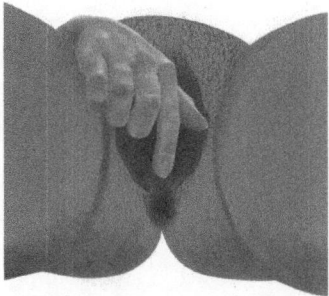

5 Prop the mirror in front of you and use one hand to gently hold open your labia minora, to see into your vagina. Check your vagina for any bumps, spots, lesions or rashes. You may see what look like 'rings' going around the vaginal wall – this is called mucosal tissue and is completely normal.

6 Finally, check your perineum (the area located between the entrance to the vagina and the anus) for any lumps, bumps or anomalies. When you have finished, wash your hands again. Make a note of any changes detected and, if you're at all worried about any anomalies, don't hesitate to consult your doctor for a professional examination.

FAIR HEALTHCARE ACCESS FOR ALL

I feel strongly that everybody – whatever their creed, colour, background, ability or gender expression – should have equal access to healthcare when they visit my surgery or any other service in the healthcare system.

However, this is still not the case for many people trying to access healthcare and advice. Patients can be discriminated against for many reasons and access to fair healthcare for ethnic minorities, those who are disabled and the LGBTQ+ community is woefully below the ideal standard. In order to counterbalance this, and to ensure that such disparity and discrimination is eradicated, we need allies to help fight our corner, and ambassadors to try to connect with our communities.

ETHNIC MINORITIES

Institutional racism and systemic misogyny continue to prevail in healthcare, to the detriment of ethnic minority women. The health issues of women of colour are often dismissed by clinicians or their own community, and their pain is downplayed and invalidated.

In some ethnic minority communities, when someone is unwell they're more likely to have a mindset of 'I will be cured if I pray hard enough' or 'this is a test of my faith'. This can lead to a reticence to address any symptoms with a doctor, and the shame and stigma persists. Women are also less likely to discuss women's health matters with others in their community – whether that's talking about examining themselves, or about a lump they've found – and this inhibits vital information sharing. It's really important for us to recognize this issue within ethnic minority communities, and to realize that more health advocates are needed in situ to raise awareness and strengthen messages.

I'm all too aware that, among Black and Asian ethnic minorities, there's still a lot of shame and stigma around breast examinations, for example. Within some parts of society – particularly faith-based communities – breasts are highly sexualized, prompting the mindset that they're something to keep hidden. This often deters women from checking their breasts at home, or having them examined by a doctor. Whatever their symptoms, ethnic minority women are also more likely to wait for an appointment with a female doctor which, due to sheer demand, can lead to a delay. If you have an immediate health concern you may be seen much quicker by a male doctor, who will be more than happy to offer you a chaperone, or let a friend or family member accompany you.

When you make a medical appointment, don't be afraid to state your preferences:

- If you feel uncomfortable being seen by a doctor of a particular gender, you may state your preference to the receptionist.
- Ask to bring someone with you to your appointment (a friend or family member) or, alternatively, you can put in an advance request for the surgery to provide a chaperone; this might be another health professional.

All doctor's surgeries will offer you a chaperone during an appointment if you prefer, or will let you take a friend or family member with you.

If English isn't your first language, and none of the doctors happen to speak your first language, you can ask the receptionist to book an interpreter for you or, if you prefer, take someone to the appointment who can translate for you.

Removing barriers

Language can be a significant obstacle for women whose mother tongue is Urdu or Punjabi, for example, and who are unable to see a doctor who speaks it. Talking about menopause or other women's health issues can be embarrassing enough for these patients, but saying 'my night sweats soak my sheets' or 'sex with my husband is really painful' via a family chaperone or an interpreter can be problematic. In order to address these issues, not only do we need a more ethnically diverse workforce in the healthcare sector, we also need Western-trained doctors (myself included) to recognize these cultural barriers.

A lack of understanding about women's health can prevent ethnic minority women from accessing the care they need. It's become a personal mission of mine to target more evidence-based information at these hard-to-reach communities, and I regularly post short videos and longer-form interviews and Q&As on social media. Most of my posts on TikTok, Twitter and Instagram are spoken or subtitled in Urdu and Punjabi, as I've realized that many women in those communities will respond much better to verbal rather than written information (illiteracy levels are particularly high among first-generation South Asian female migrants). My social media feeds share the same handle – @DrNighatArif – so please feel free to watch and share.

> If English isn't your first language, you can ask for a translator if necessary (although you may have to be quite insistent).

Improving representation

Most healthcare-related promotional material – including many leaflets, posters and illustrations – does not feature people of colour. This can send the wrong message to ethnic minorities who feel excluded from mainstream medicine and are less likely to engage with healthcare professionals.

I'm doing my utmost to try to change this. In 2019 I worked with the Pausitivity campaign group to produce a #KnowYourMenopause poster in Urdu, specifically aimed at connecting with midlife women in South Asian communities. Being the first of its kind, the poster had a massive impact when it was distributed to doctors' surgeries and community centres across the UK. A poster was also produced in Welsh, too.

Over the last few years I've also had the privilege of appearing on TV including the BBC and ITV to discuss medical matters, often from a women's health perspective, which range from hot flushes to vaginal dryness. The response from my South Asian sisters has been overwhelmingly positive. They appreciate watching someone on TV who speaks for them and looks like them; let's be honest, there aren't many Muslim women wearing pink hijabs on national TV! There's no doubt about it . . . representation matters.

8.9% of residents of England and Wales did not have English as their main language in 2021

ETHNIC MINORITIES

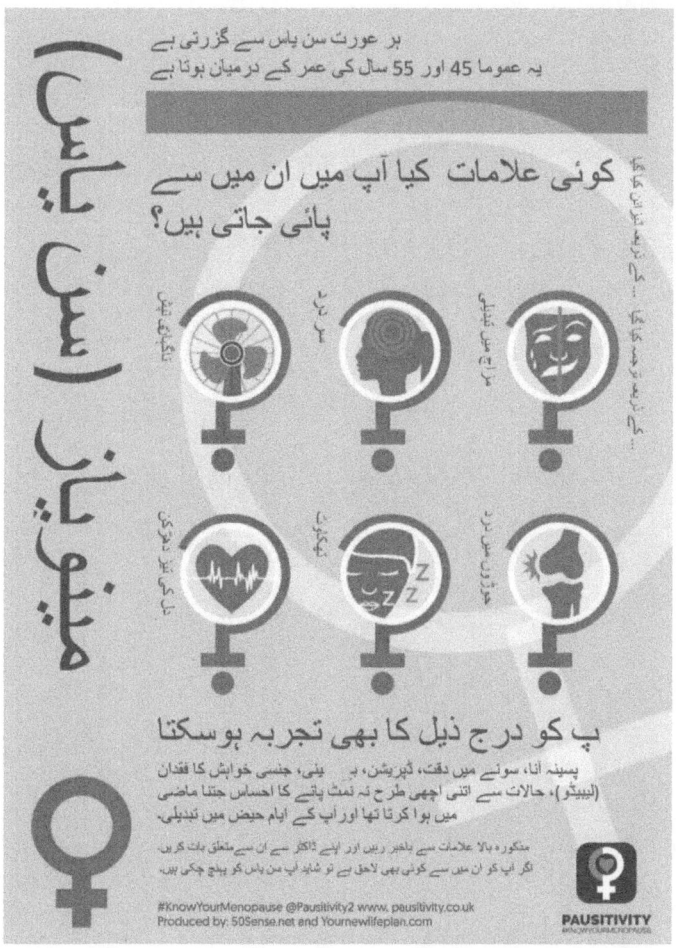

My 2019 collaboration with Pausitivity, which produced posters in Urdu to raise awareness of menopause symptoms in the South Asian community. The Pausitivity team also produced a Welsh-language poster to increase awareness in Welsh-speaking communities. Posters reproduced with thanks to Elizabeth Carr-Ellis and the Pausitivity team.

WOMEN'S HEALTH & DISABILITY

In order to reduce barriers to healthcare, doctors should make their surgeries and consultations as accessible as possible, and we should be acting as ambassadors and allies for all patients.

A 2021 article entitled 'Barriers in access to healthcare for women with disabilities' in the *BMC Women's Health* journal stated that 'women with disabilities (WWD) are more likely to have unmet healthcare needs than women without disabilities'. This statement was corroborated by the following findings outlined by the Sisters of Frida organization, a collective of disabled women:

- Disabled women have limited access to prenatal care and reproductive health services.
- Most maternity care does not meet the needs of disabled women.
- Disabled, older, asylum-seeking and Traveller women face obstacles in accessing healthcare.

In my own practice, I strive to ensure that all of my patients with physical disabilities receive the same healthcare as my able-bodied patients, and I will consider certain practicalities, such as adapting the way I fit a wheelchair user with a coil, or discussing which period products might suit their circumstances. I'll always outline the risks and benefits to an individual so they are in total control of their decision; empowering my patients is what I'm here for! If a patient is visually impaired, I'll often record voice notes, instead of writing things down or printing things out.

I also tend to use audio-based instructions for anyone who has difficulties with reading; summarizing their contraceptive options via voice notes on their phone, for instance, will always optimize healthcare for these people more than a factsheet or website. Patients with hearing loss are welcome to attend my consultations with a British Sign Language (BSL) interpreter. This is often a friend or family member but outside of this, the options are sadly limited. (A free remote interpreting service – BSL Health Access – was set up in 2020 to enable deaf people to access phone consultations but, at the time of writing, is sadly no longer funded.) Clarity of communication is vitally important when you're discussing life-changing decisions, and I hope this barrier will be removed soon.

Consultations can also be complex if I'm seeing a patient with a cognitive impairment, perhaps associated with a condition like Down's syndrome or Huntington's disease, or with neurodiverse conditions. In these instances, the way in which I communicate their healthcare options, and the way I obtain medical consent, often has to be adjusted. While I'll endeavour to involve the patient as much as possible, if they are unable to make cognitive decisions about fertility or contraception, for example, I may choose to consult with the person who has the patient's best interests at heart and who can make a decision on their behalf, often a parent, sibling or guardian.

These are just some ideas for how the healthcare system can work for all, and I hope these ideas will empower you to request the adjustments *you* may need to get the best healthcare for you, and your family too.

Become your own advocate. Get informed, do your research, become empowered and DO NOT accept discriminatory behaviour.

RIGHTS FOR TRANS PATIENTS
(& ADVICE FOR THEIR DOCTORS)

Fear and apprehension can often deter trans people from seeing their doctor. This is a heart-breaking situation that can have potentially harmful consequences.

The 2018 Stonewall *LGBT in Britain Health Report* stated that, while there are 'committed individuals and organizations doing outstanding work' in the NHS and beyond, it is also true that 'instances of discrimination, hostility and unfair treatment in healthcare services are still commonplace'. Indeed, three in five trans people (62 per cent) said they'd experienced a lack of understanding of specific trans health needs by healthcare staff.

In 2021, the TransActual organization conducted their Trans Lives survey, a cross-sectional study that recorded the experiences of trans people, including those of colour and those with disabilities. Their findings were truly depressing. Fourteen per cent of respondents had been refused medical care on at least one occasion, on account of being trans. Fifty-seven per cent of trans people – that's more than half – said they had avoided going to the doctor when unwell. Fifty-three per cent of trans people of colour experienced racism while accessing trans-specific healthcare services, and 60 per cent of disabled respondents reported suffering ableism in similar circumstances.

So how can the GP experience be improved for trans

patients? Luckily, significant steps are possible to overcome those barriers and optimize their healthcare and the majority of healthcare professionals are inclusive and supportive of such adaptations and changes. The following advice, I hope, will be helpful to both patients *and* clinicians.

Changing your name & gender details

Any patient can change their name and gender on their doctor's medical records, and this can be done as an informal decision for those under the age of 16 (before they can legally change their name via deed poll). An individual can also state their preferred pronouns, whether it's he/him, she/her or they/them, for example. Surgeries should have a specific form for this purpose, which can usually be provided by the admin team. Your details will be updated on the practice IT network, and will appear on your doctor's computer screen, so there should be no need to 'explain' yourself at an appointment, which can be upsetting. More recently I've got into the habit of asking all my patients to confirm their preferred pronouns; I think it's quite an empowering thing to do.

Surgery trans policy

Ideally, your surgery will have a trans health policy and, even better, a practitioner who has a specialist interest in trans healthcare who will be best placed to understand your emotional and physical needs. For those doctors who feel their knowledge is lacking in this area – or needs updating – there are many opportunities for further learning and continual professional development and I'd like to encourage all doctors (and people!) to be aware of trans issues and how they can affect the individuals concerned.

Routine cancer screening

When a trans person changes their gender details, they are often issued with a new NHS number. It's really important to obtain confirmation from the doctor's surgery that your data has been migrated successfully so that you'll continue to receive invites for national cancer screening programmes.

Trans men, trans women and non-binary people aged 50-plus should receive an invite for a mammogram if they have breast tissue (due to either naturally occurring oestrogen or oestrogen hormone replacement). A trans man with a uterus will need to attend a cervical smear test every three years between the ages of 25 and 49, and every five years after that until they are 65.

Trans people who've changed their gender marker may not necessarily receive automatic call and recall invites for the relevant cancer screenings so please check that you've not been missed off any lists by flagging this with your healthcare provider. Ideally, there should be a member of staff with sole responsibility for keeping track of the trans patients in the recall system; my own practice has a nurse dedicated to that very task.

It's vital that trans people don't miss out on cancer screening. Double-check with your doctor that you're in the system.

Gender identity clinic referral

I hear many cases of trans people being met with ignorance, even hostility, when they've requested a referral to a gender identity, or gender dysphoria clinic (GDC), perhaps to access gender-specific counselling, medical or surgical affirming therapy, or hormone therapy. This situation requires specialist care, and patients should expect to be treated with dignity and respect before being signposted accordingly (see pages 171–2 for referral options). There is also plenty of valuable guidance for doctors on the General Medical Council website, including shared care agreements and bridging prescriptions.

Shared care agreements

Some adult trans people (those over the age of 18) choose to access private healthcare for their hormone therapy – often because the waiting list for NHS clinics is so long (often years rather than months). I advise anyone doing this to diligently keep notes of your treatment as, by pursuing the private route, you are in effect becoming your own caregiver (you'll have to monitor your own blood hormone levels, for example).

You can, however, ask your GP to draw up a 'shared-care agreement' that allows an exchange of information between your private clinic and your doctor's surgery. Having these notes to hand will enable your GP to help with any issues associated with your hormone therapy, such as disrupted menstruation, clitoral growth, increased libido, increased facial and body hair (for trans men); or reduced facial and body hair, lower libido, decreased sexual function and genital shrinkage (for trans women).

Bridging prescriptions

In certain circumstances, adult trans patients who are waiting for treatment at a gender identity clinic can benefit from 'bridging' prescriptions. General Medical Council guidance currently allows GPs (preferably in collaboration with the gender identity clinic) to prescribe hormone treatment to patients who are suffering physically and/or psychologically as they wait for an appointment. In normal circumstances – outside of the bridging prescription remit – GPs are not usually expected to prescribe hormones to trans people unless they have the expertise and knowledge required.

As this has no impact on NHS budgets – hormones are relatively cheap, after all – many clinicians see this as discriminatory. My fellow GP, Dr Kamilla Kamaruddin, is a passionate advocate for trans health and is among those who find this situation problematic. When we last caught up she questioned the fact that GPs could give hormone treatment to cisgender males who had hypogonadism (a condition that can cause erectile dysfunction), the safety profile for which is similar to prescribing testosterone treatment to trans-masculine people, and GPs could also prescribe gonadotropin-releasing hormones to cisgender male patients with prostate cancer, and to cisgender females with endometriosis, but some GPs were reluctant to prescribe hormones to trans patients under a shared-care prescribing agreement with the GDC.

Complaints procedure

Each surgery has a complaints procedure. If you experience any form of intolerance or discrimination from a doctor, or a member of surgery staff, or if your GP has done nothing to help you, you should report it. You can either register a complaint with your practice manager or contact your local health authority (this advice applies to patients across the board, of course). You are also entitled to request to see a different doctor within your practice, and you can switch your surgery without having to provide a reason. Your local LGBTQ+ group may be able to suggest a more suitable alternative.

When people gain useful knowledge and information about their health issues, they'll go around sprinkling it like confetti . . .

PUBERTY & PERIODS

INTRODUCTION

Girls reach puberty as early as age nine or as late as seventeen, and for many it can be an uncomfortable and disconcerting time. Alongside all the changes that the body undergoes, there's a whole host of emotions and mental health considerations that can make young women feel like they're on a rollercoaster at times. If this is you right now, then I want to take this opportunity to congratulate you on starting this new phase of life. You are becoming more grown up and independent.

I know this stage can feel overwhelming, but I believe that arming yourself with the knowledge of what your body is going through, what to expect (and the huge variations of 'normal' that are possible) and when you should seek additional advice is a really important part of growing up. In this book, I'll talk you through the changes your body will undergo during puberty, as well as the practicalities of dealing with your period and contraception, for when you are ready. In addition, I'll cover issues, both mental and physical, that can arise during your monthly cycle, as well as possible infections and sexually transmitted diseases (STDs), and how they are treated.

ADVICE FOR PARENTS & CARERS

While I'm very keen for this book to help women and girls understand their bodies, I'm just as keen to inform and educate their loved ones (so that means mums, dads, siblings, grandparents or any other carers or relatives).

I'm especially keen to inform single fathers, or those in same-sex relationships, who don't have a female partner with whom to discuss women's health issues. It's so important that you are able to discuss your daughter's health with her openly.

For starters, parents and carers need to learn to use proper anatomical terms for female genitalia instead of resorting to silly euphemisms. It's a real bugbear of mine. Talking about 'tuppences', 'foo-foos' and 'front bottoms' is not helpful to anyone, and can be really confusing and misleading for a young child (and pretty cringe-worthy for an older child). If we, as the grown-ups in the room, are going to have sensible and practical conversations with our young people about periods and puberty, we need to rid ourselves of the mindset that using anatomical terms is somehow vulgar and inappropriate. It really isn't; in fact, I'd say the opposite is true. So I urge all parents and carers to ditch the daft nicknames and get into the habit of talking about vulvas and vaginas with your children, from their toddler years to their teenage years. Perhaps refer to the illustrations on pages 11–17 as a guide to using the correct genital terminology.

Educating boys about all aspects of women's health is an incredibly important part of their upbringing, in my view. Most live with women who menstruate or are going through perimenopause, such as their mum, sister or grandmother, yet the subject of women's health is rarely discussed. The boys and men in the household can only benefit from factual information to help them understand these natural bodily functions.

For instance, if you're a parent and your four-year-old spots a tampon in the bathroom and asks what it is, don't just pretend you haven't heard and change the subject. Be honest with him. Use clear and simple language. You could perhaps say, 'Women bleed a little from their vaginas every month. It's called a period. It isn't because they've hurt themselves, it's how their body gets ready in case it needs to make a baby. This is called a tampon. It catches the blood so it doesn't go onto their underwear.' I'm a huge fan of plain and honest speaking!

PHYSICAL CHANGES DURING PUBERTY

Puberty is a time of significant change: your emotions will be in flux and your body will undergo significant changes. But it is an exciting time as you change from being a child to preparing for adulthood!

Each person experiences the physical changes of puberty at a different rate and there's no specific order, so don't worry if your friend has developed breasts but you haven't. Your time will come! Here are some details of what will change:

- **Breasts** will develop and grow, and not always at the same rate as one another, so it is completely normal to have one breast bigger than the other. Developing breasts can feel quite tender. As your breasts start to develop it's a good idea to get fitted for a comfortable bra or support top. See pages 25–9 for more details.
- **Height** can increase suddenly as you experience growth spurts during puberty, or you may grow more gradually than your peers.
- **Body shape** can become more rounded, especially around the waist, hips and legs.
- **Hair** will develop in your armpits and pubic region, and the rest of your body hair (on your arms and legs in particular) may become thicker.
- **Sweat** increases in volume through puberty and it might be the first time you notice yourself sweating.

This can cause body odour so keeping clean and fresh is important.
- **Vaginal discharge** is a thin, clear or whiteish fluid that you may notice in your knickers. This is a natural secretion and helps to keep your vagina healthy and prevents infection.
- **Skin** can feel dryer or oilier as hormone levels fluctuate. You may experience outbreaks of spots either around your period or through the month. Acne is a more serious and persistent outbreak of spots that can last beyond puberty. Seek help from your doctor if you would like to explore ways to control spots and acne.
- **Periods** are a sign that your uterus is preparing for reproduction (although it may be decades before you decide to have children, if you ever do!). They result in a monthly bleed and there are a range of period products that you can choose to use during this time (see pages 78–87).

PERIODS

Did you know that women, on average, have 500 periods in their lifetime? That's around 12 per year for around 40 years. However, despite being a normal and natural part of life, periods remain a taboo subject. Many women and girls still don't feel able to speak openly about them, particularly when they have menstrual health problems such as severe pain, heavy bleeding and irregular cycles. According to a survey by Plan International UK, over half of girls in the UK have missed a day or part of a day of schooling due to their period, and around one in three women suffer from heavy menstrual bleeding that can significantly impact their daily life.

We shouldn't be made to feel embarrassed about our periods. This shame and stigma – along with a lack of awareness and education – not only harms women and girls, but also creates barriers to them seeking help. In order to change this, we all need to have more open and honest conversations about menstrual health.

The phases of your period

Your period is part of the rhythmic change of your reproductive system that is controlled by four hormones: oestrogen, progesterone, follicle stimulating hormone (FSH) and luteinizing hormone (LH). Every 28 days (on average), these hormones cleverly trigger the growth of follicles (fluid-filled sacs containing eggs in the ovaries) and prompt the release of an egg, as well as the growth and shedding of the uterus lining (the endometrium).

If an egg is not fertilized, the endometrial lining – a highly vascular tissue – comes out of the cervix and through the vagina, causing what is commonly known as a period (or menstruation). The first full day of bleeding is counted as day 1 of your menstrual cycle. This cycle comprises three separate phases, based on a 28-day cycle.

Follicular phase (days 4–14)
The oestrogen hormone triggers the release of the luteinizing hormone (LH) which, at the end of the follicular phase, causes a mature egg to be released from one of the ovaries into the corresponding fallopian tube (ovulation). You can get pregnant during this time so be aware that sperm can live inside your vagina for several days following unprotected sex.

Ovulation phase (day 14)
You can usually tell you're ovulating (releasing an egg) by a rise in your body temperature. You may notice your vaginal discharge becoming thicker, too, with a consistency similar to raw egg white. Ovulation usually happens mid-way through your cycle – around day 14 – and lasts around 24 hours. At the time of ovulation, some women can experience spotting (light traces of blood), but many others don't.

Luteal phase (days 15 onwards)

In this stage, the follicle that released its egg changes into a corpus luteum (a normal clump of cells inside your ovary that forms during each period). This happens immediately after the egg leaves the ovary at ovulation. The corpus luteum releases oestrogen and progesterone. Both these hormones are associated with premenstrual syndrome (PMS, see page 106) which can cause symptoms such as bloating, fatigue, irritability and tearfulness.

If your egg is fertilized in this phase, the progesterone hormone will support early pregnancy. But if it's not fertilized, the corpus luteum will begin to break down, usually about 9–11 days after ovulation. This results in a drop in oestrogen and progesterone levels, which ultimately causes menstruation. The lining of the uterus (the endometrium) secretes chemicals that will either help an early pregnancy or break down the lining – this phase can also be known as the secretory phase.

13% of UK schoolgirls miss a day of school every month due to their period

Starting your periods

Typically, you will begin your periods about two years after your breasts start developing and, on average, about two years after you notice a white vaginal discharge. Most girls will have their first period around the age of 12, but it does vary from person to person. Some girls can start menstruating when they're just eight or nine, and others can experience their first period at 14 or 15 (both of these scenarios are quite normal). However, if you or a child in your care begin menstruating at aged seven or younger – something known as 'precocious puberty' – then a visit to the doctor is in order. You should also visit your doctor if you haven't had a period by the age of 16.

EGG → FERTILIZED = PREGNANCY

EGG NOT FERTILIZED → BREAKDOWN OF THE LINING OF THE UTERUS = BLEEDING

Endometrial lining & follicle development during your cycle

The endometrial lining breaks down from day 1 of your cycle and is expelled through the vagina. Once shed, the endometrium will thicken through the follicular phase, ovulation and the early luteal phase. At the same time one follicle in one ovary will mature until an egg is ready for release (ovulation), then the egg travels down the fallopian tube and into the uterus. The empty follicle will then close. If the released egg is fertilized then it will attempt to embed in the thickened endometrial lining of the uterus.

PERIODS

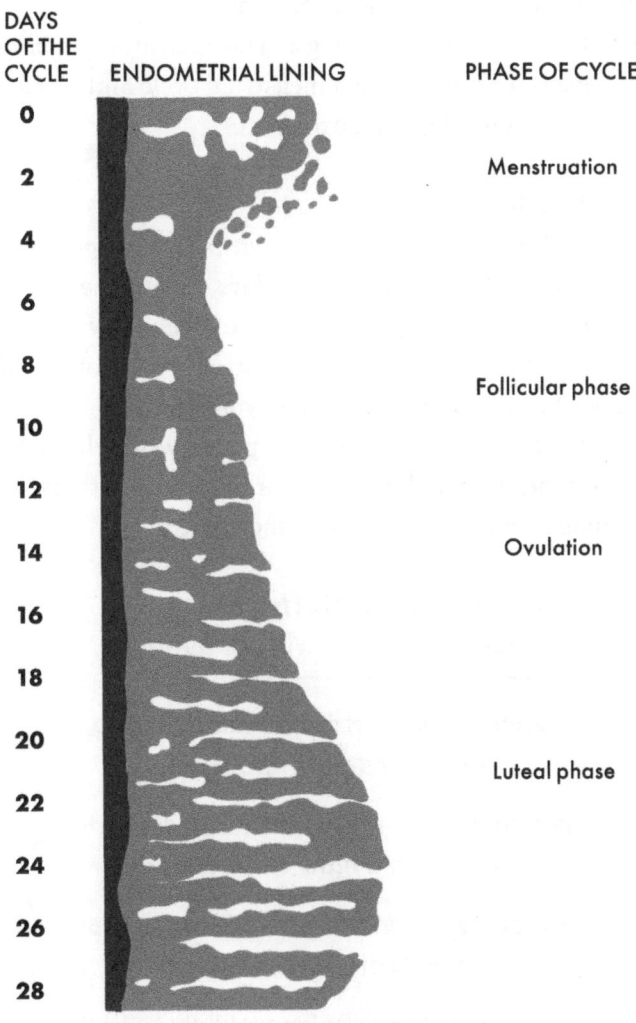

What to expect from your period
In real life there is no such thing as a normal, average period. Everyone is different, with a menstrual cycle and bleeding pattern that is totally unique to them.

Period length
The length of a period differs from person to person. It usually lasts between five and six days, but can be as short as two to four days, or as long as eight to twelve days. Ideally, though, you need to view your menstrual cycle holistically, instead of just focusing on the days you bleed.

Understanding each different phase will help you to pinpoint the ups and downs of your mood and activity, and to manage your life and routines more effectively.

It's perfectly fine to ask yourself the following questions:

When is the best time of my cycle to make a serious decision?

Which days would be more suitable for me to train hard in the gym?

Which weekend am I more likely to feel confident and outgoing?

Which weekend am I more likely to feel irritable and antisocial?

FACT:
a 'normal' period doesn't exist; we all have different cycles

Familiarizing yourself with your menstrual cycle, from start to finish, can be a really useful way to identify your physical and emotional peaks and troughs.

Period regularity
Most medical textbooks will state the average menstrual cycle as being 28 days but, from my clinical experience, anything between 21 and 40 days is quite normal if it follows a regular pattern. However, girls who have just started their periods can have very irregular cycles at first – it takes a while for the body to settle into a routine – but if this continues for 12 to 24 months, please do book an appointment to see your doctor.

A woman's menstrual cycle may become irregular for a variety of reasons. Certain conditions can cause the cycle to change – such as fibroids (see page 179), endometriosis (see page 179) and polycystic ovary syndrome (PCOS, see page 183) – and periods may become quite erratic up to eight years before a woman reaches menopause and they stop.

Diet and stress can also have an impact on your menstrual cycle. Sudden or excessive weight loss can cause your periods to become irregular or stop altogether, because the body isn't healthy enough to support a pregnancy. If you have excessive weight gain, the fat cells in your body may produce an increased amount of oestrogen hormone, which can cause periods to become irregular or stop entirely. When we feel stressed, anxious or worried, our body goes into fight-or-flight mode due to a rush of adrenaline and increased cortisol (a steroid hormone). This in turn affects the hormones that trigger ovulation, which can cause disruption to your menstrual cycle. Stress can prompt an early period, irregular periods, late periods or can stop your periods altogether – sometimes for several months.

Period colour & consistency
The colour of your menstrual blood will change as your period progresses; you might notice that it's brownish at the beginning and end of your bleed, and bright red in the middle.

The consistency and texture of your discharge will also vary, from thin and watery on day 1, perhaps, to thick and sticky on day 3.

Flow and volume will change, too; you may only require a 'regular' pad or tampon in the early stages of your period when your flow is light, but may need to increase it to 'super' as your flow becomes heavier. Remember, these changes are all unique to each unique person.

The changes to your flow

The volume, colour and texture of menstrual blood will change over your period. Often it will appear a little lumpy and darker at the start (as small clots from the endometrium lining fall away), turning more uniform and bright red before getting lighter in volume and colour towards the end of your period.

Start of period
Heavier flow/thicker texture

End of period
Lighter flow/thinner texture

Tracking your period

From the moment you start your periods, you should begin tracking your cycle. It's a great piece of advice that I dish out to all my patients who menstruate. By keeping a record of your cycle from one month to the next, you'll get a really clear idea of your own unique pattern.

You can track your cycle by simply jotting things down in a diary or, even better, by downloading a free period tracking app onto your phone. I really can't recommend these apps enough; they're such handy little tools and are so simple to use. See the Resources section (on page 187) for more information.

Having this information to hand during a medical

appointment can be extremely useful. Assessing your tracking data will help your doctor to gauge whether your cycle is imbalanced or out of sync, and will give them a much better idea of the symptoms you're experiencing and the treatment you require.

Things to monitor
- Date your period starts and stops Blood flow (low to high)
- Blood consistency (thin to thick)
- Physical symptoms (stomach cramps, headaches)
- Emotional symptoms (irritability, tearfulness)

PERIODS

NOTES ON MY PERIOD

DAY 1
Cried at a nature programme today! Then found I'd started my period just before I went to bed.

DAY 2
Feeling teary on and off for much of the day. Also had stomach cramps and ache in vulva. Heavy flow with some clots.

DAY 3
Stomach cramps and vulva ache continued but mood much better. Flow still heavy.

DAY 4
Flow lighter today and cramps and vulva ache have gone. Feeling pretty tired so went to bed early.

DAY 5
Light flow and a couple of spots appeared on my chin.

DAY 6
Very light, pink spotting today.

Period products

During their lifetime, most women will get through between 14,000 and 18,000 disposable pads, liners or tampons. There's a huge range of period products on the market these days, and deciding which type or brand best suits you can seem very daunting when you first start your periods. It's often a case of trial and error, as well as personal preference – some people choose reusable products, some choose single-use products; some people choose pads, some choose tampons, and others use a combination of both – but it should be based on what you like, what you feel comfortable with, and what you can afford or have access to.

Always read the instructions on your period products, so you know you're using them correctly, and bear in mind that leaks can occasionally occur with any type of period product. Make a habit of changing your period product regularly – every four hours or so (or each time you pass urine) is a good rule of thumb for tampons and pads. Period cups can usually last a little longer, but ensure you give them a proper clean in the sink under clean running water when you empty it and reinsert.

Which period products should you choose?

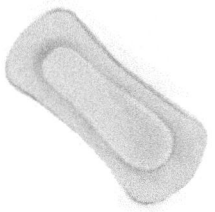

Pads without wings
Worn inside your pants and held in place with a sticky strip.

Pros
- Different shapes and sizes for different flows.
- Easy to apply to pants.

Cons
- Can leak at the sides.
- Can shift about in your pants.
- Can be bulky to carry around in your bag.
- Can't swim in them.
- Can't wear a thong.
- Single use so not as environmentally friendly as reusable options.

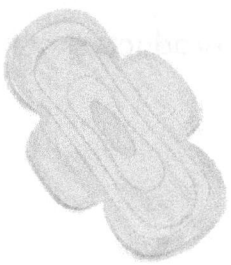

Pads with wings
Worn inside your pants and held in place with a sticky strip and side flaps.

Pros
- Different shapes and sizes for different flows.
- More secure in your pants than pads without wings.
- Less chance of leaking compared to pads without wings.

Cons
- Can leak if wrong absorbency is chosen.
- Wings can cause chafing in the groin and thighs as they rub.
- Can be bulky to carry around in your bag.
- Can't swim in them.
- Can't wear a thong.
- Single use so not as environmentally friendly as reusable options.

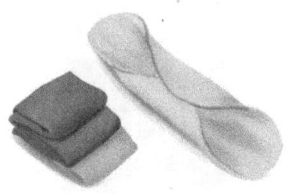

Reusable pads
Worn inside your pants and held in place with popper fastenings.

Pros
- Reusable, so more environmentally friendly and cost-effective in the long term.
- Different shapes and sizes for different flows.
- Easy to apply to pants.

Cons
- Bulky to carry around in your bag.
- Will need to carry a waterproof bag for used pads if you are on the go.
- Can't swim in them.
- Can't wear a thong.

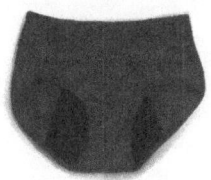

Period pants
Underwear with additional absorbency in the gusset to keep you dry.

Pros
- Reusable, so more environmentally friendly and cost-effective in the long term.
- Different sizes and styles for different flows.
- Can also be used alongside internal protection (period cup or tampon) for extra peace of mind on heavier days.
- Sometimes also available as a swimwear version, so you can wear during swimming.

Cons
- More costly than regular underwear.
- Can be bulky to carry around in your bag if your flow is heavy and you are out for the whole day; carry a waterproof bag and a spare in case you need to change.

PERIODS

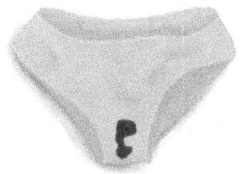

Free bleeding
Not wearing period 'protection' and allowing menstrual blood to flow freely.

Pros
- Can bleed as nature intended.
- No products, so environmentally friendly.
- Has been practised for millennia and more recently used as a protest about taxes on period products, disposable period products and silencing of women's issues.

Cons
- No protection, so can cause stains on clothing, seating and bedlinen.
- Can increase your laundry load.

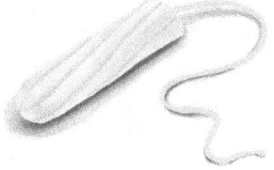

Tampons

A soft tube that is inserted into the vagina with an applicator or finger.

Pros
- Different absorbencies to suit flow.
- Discreet; can fit in the palm, and purse or pocket.
- Can be worn while swimming.
- The external string isn't visible once inserted.
- Can't feel the tampon once it's inside.
- Can wear with a thong.

Cons
- Can leak if wrong absorbency is chosen.
- Very rarely can cause toxic shock syndrome (TSS), easily prevented if changed regularly.
- Inserting a tampon can sometimes be uncomfortable (especially the first time).
- If incorrectly inserted, it can be expelled from the vaginal canal.
- Single use so not as environmentally friendly as reusable options.

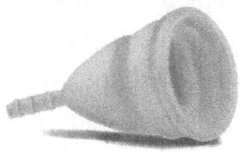

Period cup
A soft cup that is folded and inserted into the vagina to collect blood.

Pros
- Reusable, so more environmentally friendly and cost-effective in the long term.
- Can be left in for up to eight hours before taking out and rinsing.
- Some versions can be worn during sex.
- Can be worn while swimming.
- Can't feel the cup once it's inside.
- Can wear with a thong.

Cons
- Insertion can be tricky; it needs practice.
- Can be messy; you have to use your finger to fish it out before rinsing.
- Needs a thorough wash after use.
- If you have heavy flow the cup can overflow.
- If you have fibroids the cup can get in the way and be uncomfortable.

Period products for trans & non-binary people

Much more work needs to be done by manufacturers to make period products more inclusive for trans and non-binary people who menstruate. Most pads, pants and tampons are sold in feminine-looking packaging (so lots of pink flowers, birds and butterflies) that, according to patients I speak with, can trigger their dysphoria (see page 168) and make them feel uncomfortable when purchasing them in shops. Because of this, many trans and non-binary people resort to buying their products online, often opting for period pants with plain designs, or period cups with gender-neutral packaging.

Period products & the environment

Did you know that we all have our own period mountains? I used to think that liners, pads and tampon applicators were incinerated, but this isn't always the case; most of them are left sitting on our beautiful planet. I was horrified to hear from a green-minded colleague that each packet of pads contains the equivalent of four plastic bags (and we all know how long that would take to decompose).

If you can, I'd really recommend that you consider trying reusable period products like the pads, pants and cups. The initial outlay may prove to be more expensive than disposable products, but in the long term it works out more cost-effective because they can last for years. And, since they're more sustainable than disposable period products, they're much better for the environment.

If you do use disposable period products, don't flush them down the toilet. Please bin them sensibly. Don't wrap a used pad in a plastic bag or reams of toilet paper because you're worried someone will see it; just roll it up and pop it in the bin.

Period products & sport
It's quite normal for women and girls to stay active or play sport when they're menstruating. Some may prefer not to do so, which is totally fine – they could have very heavy flow, or bad period pain, and might want to take it easy – but others may find that exercise makes them feel better during their period, both physically and emotionally. For reasons of comfort and practicality, most women who participate in sport prefer to use tampons (especially if they're swimming or cycling) or reusable period-proof swimwear or shorts, but pads are perfectly suitable for low-intensity forms of exercise such as walking or Pilates.

A year's worth of disposable period products contributes 5.3kg of CO_2

PERIOD INEQUALITY

Period inequality is an unequal access to period products, education and menstrual care because of boundaries of economics, ethnicity or culture. It is vital that women everywhere, regardless of their race or class, are able to access the period products and knowledge they need to experience their period each month without it impacting their work, education or home life.

A survey conducted in 2019 by Plan International highlighted that one in ten girls in the UK could not afford period products. During the Coronavirus pandemic this figure went up to one in three.

Some people use the expression 'period poverty' to describe the struggle faced by women who cannot access safe and affordable products. I find this terminology incredibly demeaning, and prefer not to use it. Firstly, if you can't afford food or you belong to a low-income household, the last thing you want to be labelled as is suffering from 'period poverty'. Secondly, it suggests that women are weak, powerless victims of their periods, and that this perfectly natural process is a hardship or a hindrance. Thirdly, it also belittles the deep inequality and discrimination they face in these circumstances, which often stems from race, class, gender or socio-economic status.

This pejorative terminology also implies that this problem is largely confined to developing countries, which simply isn't true. Period product inequality is a global issue – UK food banks frequently appeal for donations of pads and tampons for low-income women – and it has serious repercussions. Limited access to period products can deter girls from attending school, or women from attending work, thus restricting their educational and professional development, and earning power and opportunities. Using alternative 'protection' (like rags or toilet tissue) can lead to harmful infection and the associated blood leakages can cause shame and embarrassment.

I find it all so saddening and infuriating. Governments around the world need to get a better grip on the situation, and work more closely with women's health organizations, if we're going to put an end to this unfairness. With that in mind, my good friend Manjit Gill MBE founded Binti International, an organization that seeks to provide menstrual dignity to girls around the world (their mantra is 'availability, affordability and awareness'). She talks of the necessity of a 'period revolution' to normalize menstruation and to eradicate stigma and suffering, and has led a campaign for all business and public spaces to have free period products.

If you're having problems accessing period products, please don't suffer in silence. Speak to a health professional who may be able to signpost you to an organization that can help, or see Resources on page 187.

LET'S TALK ABOUT PERIODS

Periods are a natural and completely normal element of puberty and beyond and as a society we need to be more open about discussions around them – not just between women, but between men, women, trans and non-binary people.

While this book aims to help women and girls understand their periods, I can't emphasize enough that it's also so important for *everyone* close to them, including single dads or those in same-sex relationships, to feel comfortable talking about periods with their daughters, and that they can deal with the subject openly, honestly and without embarrassment.

The good news is that attitudes among fathers could well be changing. A YouGov survey commissioned by the charity Action Aid in 2017, to mark Menstrual Hygiene Day, revealed that while nearly half (47 per cent) of daughters said they'd feel uncomfortable discussing periods with their fathers, only 9 per cent of men would feel uncomfortable discussing periods with their daughters. Half of men surveyed (50 per cent) said they wouldn't feel uncomfortable buying period protection for women, yet only 16 per cent of women said they'd feel comfortable asking a man to buy period products for them. So if we're going to continue breaking down the stigma barrier, inter-generational communication is key. Daughters, talk to your dads . . . and dads, talk to your daughters!

PUBERTY & PERIODS

As far as I'm concerned, no age is off-limits when it comes to talking about menstruation. I think parents and carers should start discussing period-related matters with their children as early as possible, at a stage in their lives when they're able to absorb and understand reliable and sensible information. There's no hard and fast rule, of course – all children are different – but as a parent or carer, you'll know instinctively when the time is right to prompt that conversation. Try not to delay this too much. In many instances, the big 'period talk' when a child reaches high school age can often come much too late in the day. And please don't ignore the subject of menstruation completely, or rely on your child's teachers or classmates to tell them about it; I think we owe it to our daughters to open up that channel of communication within the family unit.

The average woman in the UK will spend up to £18,450 on products geared towards her period over a lifetime

Also, don't forget that most boys live alongside women who menstruate – their mum, their sisters and cousins, their aunts, their grandmothers – and it affects them that, all too often, periods are never discussed openly, often as a result of shame and stigma. It doesn't have to be this way, though. The males in the household cannot fail to benefit from factual, reliable information, in order that they may better understand this perfectly normal and natural bodily function.

LET'S TALK ABOUT PERIODS

When your daughter starts her periods – the average age is 12, so plan to introduce the subject at an even earlier age so she isn't surprised or confused when the time comes – it's vital that she receives support from her parents and carers. This emotional and physical milestone can be a difficult, confusing and scary time, and they will really appreciate your love and understanding. Congratulate your child on this new phase of life. Prompt a conversation by asking them how they're feeling, both physically and emotionally; whether they're getting any breast tenderness or abdominal cramps, for example, or suffering with tiredness or mood swings. Just asking your daughter about their periods is beneficial in itself; ignoring it, or just brushing it off as a 'woman's problem', is not helpful and can be quite isolating for girls who are coming to terms with their changing bodies, and who are adapting to this new phase in their lives.

There are lots of practical things you can do to help, too, not least ensuring that you have a good supply of period products for your daughter to use, or even going to the pharmacy together to buy her preferred pads or tampons. If she experiences stomach cramps, stock up the freezer with ice packs or offer to fill up a hot water bottle.

A 2017 survey revealed that nearly half of daughters in the UK said they'd feel uncomfortable discussing periods with their fathers

PUBERTY & PERIODS

If she suffers with headaches, ensure you have enough paracetamol in the bathroom cabinet. This advice applies to boyfriends, partners and husbands as well as fathers, of course. Your other halves will thank you for it!

There's plenty more you can do to help your loved one during their menstrual cycle. Try to show understanding if they're displaying tell-tale PMS signs such as tiredness, anxiety or irritability. Deal sympathetically with any instances of period blood leaking onto clothes or bedlinen, which can be quite traumatic and upsetting (and certainly seek advice from a doctor if this happens regularly). Keep school staff, or extracurricular club leaders, informed if she is suffering with period cramps, heavy flow or severe fatigue. By acting with care and compassion, you'll help to minimize those awful feelings of shame and stigma.

It's time to talk about periods . . . without shame or embarrassment!

CULTURAL ATTITUDES TOWARDS MENSTRUATION

For centuries periods have been surrounded by myths and rumours that stigmatize those who menstruate. Although improved access to education in today's society has exposed the untruth of many of these, they still prevail.

The onset of menstruation can have a huge emotional and psychological impact on a girl and a first period is seen as a significant milestone that can be associated with a 'coming of age' or 'entry into womanhood', both of which are observed communally in a Bat Mitzvah (a Jewish ritual) or a Quinceañera (a celebration in Hispanic countries that literally means 'one who is 15').

However, some communities can perceive periods as 'unclean' and as a consequence, opt to impose restrictive measures on females. In Islam, for example, women who are menstruating aren't able to pray or go to the Mosque. In Hinduism, if a woman is on her period she cannot prepare food, eat with the family or attend the temple. In some areas of rural India and Nepal, girls can be banished to customized 'period huts'. This segregation can adversely affect how a girl views her menstrual cycle, excluding her from religious events and essentially ostracizing her from her community.

In fact, a 2017 study (by the Clue period tracker app), found a remarkable number of myths and superstitions remain. In the United States many believe that using tampons might break your hymen (the thin piece of skin that partially covers your vagina) and render you 'impure' by taking away your virginal status – a ridiculous myth that is common globally. Also in the US, you (apparently) shouldn't touch vegetables during or before the pickling process because they'll go bad. And some say you can't go camping in the wild because bears will smell the blood. Totally absurd, of course, and completely untrue!

In Israel some mothers believe that slapping their daughter in the face when she gets her first period will give her beautiful red cheeks for the rest of her life. Menstruating girls are told not to shower with hot water because it will give them a heavy flow. Needless to say, there's no evidence to support either of these beliefs!

In Italy, some women stay out of the kitchen during their period because their dough won't rise properly – what nonsense! – so they won't be able to produce decent bread or pizza.

In Argentina it is said that those on their period can't make whipped cream or butter because it'll curdle. Another myth tells girls not to soak in the bath because it will cause their bleeding to stop and reduce their fertility.

In India, girls must wash their hair on the first day of menstruation in order to clean themselves but, for the remainder of their period, they are not allowed to wash their hair too much since their flow will reduce and their fertility will be affected. In fact, the link between hair and female health is very much a recurring theme in many faiths and cultures, including Islam and Judaism. A woman's 'crowning glory' is seen as a sign of beauty and a symbol of fertility, and many express the view that it shouldn't be excessively touched, washed or cut during their period. I beg to differ, of course.

And, to round things off, here are some other menstruation myths that I have come across: in Mexico, if you're on your period you should avoid vigorous dancing to active rhythms in order to protect your uterus; in Romania, you can't touch flowers because they'll die quicker; in Malaysia, you are told to wash your pads before throwing them out, otherwise ghosts will come back to haunt you; and in the Dominican Republic you can't paint your nails or drink lemonade. Washing your face with the blood from your first period gives you clear skin, according to a myth in the Philippines; and in Brazil, if you're menstruating you can't walk around barefoot otherwise you'll get bad cramps. In France, you're banned from making mayonnaise because it will curdle and, in Bolivia, you're told not to cradle babies because it will make them ill. None of these claims has an ounce of merit!

Some of these superstitions may sound bizarrely amusing, but there is a serious (and dangerous) side to all this myth-making. Many of them advocate behavioural restrictions that contribute to gender-biased taboos and discrimination. These entrenched falsehoods make it harder for girls to talk about their menstrual health and lead to shame and silence.

These myths and superstitions also push the idea that women, once they start their periods, are going to be ruining something, or restricted from doing something. Such misogynistic superstitions become embedded in certain cultures and are passed on through generations, often via mothers and grandmothers, who perpetuate them without educating their girls about the biology of their own bodies.

People need to realize, for example, that period blood is the same blood that runs through everyone's body; it just happens to incorporate the uterus lining as well as other cell matter. Too many communities believe this blood to be 'old' or 'dirty', which is wrong and misguided; if this was the case, women would have regular infections. Period blood is clean, healthy and normal.

My friend Manjit from Binti International also believes that much of the stigma and shame related to menstruation stems from its over-sexualization. Ideally, it should be taught in schools around the world as a stand-alone topic, and explained in such a way that empowers girls to understand themselves, and teaches boys to become empathetic and supportive.

There's also a misconception – one I've witnessed myself, with my own patients – that menstrual (and menopausal) matters are largely 'Western' issues that are only discussed and addressed among middle-class white women. This assumption may well stem from long-standing and deep-rooted socio-cultural attitudes and religious traditions. It may also stem from institutional failings within the healthcare system – and the fact that we still have so much to learn. But whatever the reason, it makes me feel sad and frustrated. Women and girls across the board should receive the same access to healthcare – regardless of creed, colour, class or culture – and, with that in mind, I've made it my long-term mission to help break down those barriers.

HEALTH & COMFORT ISSUES DURING YOUR MONTHLY CYCLE

Some women have trouble-free menstruation cycles that impinge little on their daily lives, but many others suffer physical or emotional issues at different times in their cycle which can have a huge impact on school, work or relationships. Here are some of the common issues.

Period pain

Period pain is no joke. It's a common but debilitating condition that should always be taken very seriously. Severe period pain is known as dysmenorrhoea and some doctors are finally admitting that period cramps can be just as painful as a heart attack, if not worse, and I think they're spot on.

So why do we get period pain, and how should we deal with it? During your menstrual period, a hormone called prostaglandin – which helps the body deal with injury and illness – causes your uterus to contract in order to expel its lining. Prostaglandin is so powerful, in fact, that it triggers labour and contractions in childbirth. When the endometrial cells lining the uterus break down the during menstruation, they also release large amounts of prostaglandin. This prostaglandin constricts the blood vessels in the uterus and makes the muscle layer constrict by causing contractions, which temporarily cut off blood supply to the uterus and starve it of oxygen. This causes a throbbing, cramping pain that can spread from your lower abdomen to your lower back. The effects of prostaglandin are localized, meaning they only act where they are produced, which is why most period pain is felt in the abdominal area.

Some women suffer a monthly host of intense physical symptoms that can include fever, nausea, inflammation, dizziness, clumsiness, tinnitus and even diarrhoea (otherwise known as 'period poops'). Having to deal with this multifactorial pain while coping with life, jobs and families makes women totally incredible, don't you think? The good news is that this release of prostaglandin is temporary and the body quickly starts to break it down, diminishing its effect on the body. This is the reason why, for the majority of women, period pain doesn't linger too long, usually straddling day 1 and day 3 of their cycle.

> We need to stop normalizing pain. Take paracetamol or ibuprofen to ease your symptoms, and if that doesn't work, see your doctor.

Painful periods:
What can you do to manage the pain?

Many women experience pain each month before and during their period. Don't be afraid to try the following solutions to manage it:

- **Take paracetamol** regularly (a maximum of two 500-milligram tablets, every four to six hours, no more than four times a day).
- **Take ibuprofen** (a maximum of two 200-milligram tablets, three times a day) in addition to paracetamol if necessary, and only if you are over 12 years old. Ibuprofen isn't tolerated by everyone though. It must only ever be taken with food – never on an empty stomach – so as not to trigger acid reflux, worsen asthma symptoms or interact with other medicines. There are other over-the-counter options containing ibuprofen lysine that are sold specifically to treat period pain, but they can be quite expensive, and you may find that generic ibuprofen does just as good a job.
- **Hot water bottles** can help to relieve cramps.
- **Drink plenty of fluids** to keep you hydrated.
- **Vitamin B1 (thiamine)** (100 milligrams daily throughout the month) can help some people.
- **Magnesium glycinate** (300–400 milligrams at bedtime, increasing to 600 milligrams for one week before a period is due) can also be beneficial.

- **Yoga** can help you to relax and relieve cramping.
- **Acupuncture** can be of great benefit to some people.
- **Quitting smoking** is good for your health anyway, but has been found to have a positive impact on period pain.
- **Cutting down on alcohol** during your period can also have a positive impact.
- **Transcutaneous electrical nerve stimulation** machines (also known as TENS) have been flagged in some data studies as having a positive effect in helping to control and regulate pain. These are available in pharmacies or online, or to hire if you would like to try before you buy.

If you find that you need to use medical pain relief during every period, and it improves your symptoms, there's nothing to be concerned about. However, if you're unable to control your period pain despite using paracetamol and/or ibuprofen, do not hesitate to see a doctor. They will assess you to pinpoint any underlying causes and will do all they can to help ease your discomfort and improve your quality of life. Do not suffer in silence. Do not 'keep calm and carry on', despite what others might tell you. Pain can be controlled, and does not have to be endured.

Premenstrual syndrome

So what is PMS, and what are its effects? During your period, hormone levels can go up and down. These hormones help your body to prepare for possible pregnancy and send signals

HEALTH & COMFORT ISSUES

back and forth between the brain and the ovaries, causing changes to the follicles and the uterus. These hormones, as they fluctuate, are responsible for premenstrual syndrome, and its troublesome symptoms include:

- Headaches and/or migraine
- Tender and/or swollen breasts
- Abdominal bloating, pain and/or cramps
- Diarrhoea and/or constipation
- Sugar cravings
- Swollen legs
- Backache
- Fluid retention
- Fatigue, lethargy and/or excessive sleepiness
- Clumsiness
- Insomnia
- Reduced libido
- Acne
- Lowered ability to cope
- Anxiety and/or nervous tension
- Anger, aggression and/or irritability
- Impairment of concentration
- Loss of confidence
- Mood swings and/or tearfulness
- Depression

Only one or two of these symptoms need to be present for a diagnosis of PMS and it is reported to be experienced by up to 50 per cent of women around the globe. Premenstrual tension

(PMT) is essentially the same condition – you'll probably hear both PMS and PMT being referred to – although most clinicians prefer to use 'syndrome' rather than 'tension' as it's a looser, more all-encompassing definition (and, some would argue, sounds a little less emotionally charged).

In terms of treatment for PMS, your doctor will be able to suggest ways you can best manage your symptoms. Emotional and psychological issues can be eased with antidepressants – selective serotonin reuptake inhibitors (SSRIs). Being prescribed with this type of medication does not necessarily mean you're suffering with depression as they're common remedies for hormonal imbalances. Long-acting reversible contraceptives (LARCS) such as implants (see page 138) and injections (see page 140) can also help to regulate your hormones.

Making changes to your routine and lifestyle can also be beneficial. I often encourage patients suffering with PMS to engage in exercise – an online yoga session, perhaps, or a walk in a park or the countryside – and, if they can, to cut out cigarettes and alcohol. Dietary supplements like vitamin B6, vitamin D, calcium and magnesium can help to improve mood and wellbeing in some cases, as can complementary therapies (I know many patients who are devotees of acupuncture, aromatherapy and reflexology, for example). Evidence with regard to alternative therapies is scant, I admit, but if something is helping someone to cope with their PMS, and is causing no harm, I'm happy for them to continue with it.

For women and girls who experience PMS, the impact on schooling, work and relationships can be significant. I've treated women whose PMS has led to exam failure, career disruption, financial losses and marriage breakdown. Yet, despite the debilitating nature of this condition, society often treats it with scorn and ridicule. Comments like, 'Is it the time of the month, love?' are woven into the fabric of many culture and it needs to stop. Sufferers need to be treated with compassion, not contempt.

Premenstrual dysphoric disorder

Premenstrual dysphoric disorder (PMDD) is a reaction in the brain to the rise and fall of oestrogen and progesterone. Symptoms can be severe and worsen over time, and can be especially prevalent around menstruation and perimenopause. PMDD symptoms can also be felt around times of pregnancy, birth and miscarriage, despite the absence of menstrual bleeds. It is a worse extension of PMS, and sometimes can be disabling.

The International Association for Premenstrual Disorders (IAPMD) states that a diagnosis of PMDD must include one of the five core symptoms:

- Emotional changes, such as extreme mood swings, tearfulness, sudden extreme sadness or increased sensitivity to rejection, which can disrupt daily life and damage relationships
- Irritability and/or anger, perhaps including increased conflict with family and friends
- Depressed mood, or suicidal thoughts
- Feeling hopeless or worthless

- Anxiety and tension, or feelings of being on edge or 'keyed up'

A PMDD diagnosis should also include the presence of at least five of these symptoms:

- Difficulty concentrating, focusing, or thinking; brain fog
- Decreased interest in usual activities (work, school, friends, hobbies)
- Tiredness or low energy
- Food cravings, overeating or changes in appetite
- Bloating or weight gain
- Insomnia
- Feeling out of control
- Breast tenderness
- Joint or muscle pain

PMDD is diagnosed by tracking symptoms and these should be recorded daily for at least two menstrual cycles (again, yet another good reason to track your periods – see page 75). There is also a 'self-screen' test available on the IAPMD website (see Resources on page 187) that allows you to input your symptoms. Taking the resulting data to your healthcare appointment would be extremely helpful.

PMDD can be treated with SSRI antidepressants, the combined oral contraceptive pill, or gonadotropin-releasing hormone analogues (GnRHa) that involve monthly injections to manage the condition. Ovulation suppressants such as transdermal oestrogen or cyclical progesterone can help, as can cognitive behavioural therapy (CBT). In some circumstances an abdominal hysterectomy (the removal of the uterus) will be necessary.

I fear there's a lack of understanding regarding PMDD among some healthcare professionals, and there's no doubt that more medical research is needed as there is emerging evidence that those who have PMDD, or PMS, may experience heightened symptoms if they are neurodiverse. The IAPMD website contains an extensive treatment plan that people and clinicians can familiarize themselves with and, on a larger scale, I'm hoping that more detailed studies will be commissioned to discover more about this debilitating condition.

Food cravings

So why do we have food cravings just before or during our periods? During the luteal phase (when an ovary has released an egg, before our period starts) we experience a fluctuation in hormones, which often includes a dip in serotonin levels. Sometimes referred to as the 'happy hormone', serotonin is a chemical that can help to control appetite, sleep, sexual desire, body temperature and social behaviour. Eating carbohydrates (so that's broadly sugary, starchy and fibre-based foods) serves to boost these serotonin levels, hence why those PMS sufferers who feel tired and tetchy will find themselves reaching out for bread, biscuits and chocolate bars!

I don't have a massive problem with people satisfying their carb cravings, within reason (as a cake-lover myself, the occasional slice of Victoria sponge never fails to cheer me up if I'm feeling low!). However, to counterbalance the odd lapse – and to help keep your cravings under control – try to choose a varied and balanced diet that's rich in fruit, vegetables, whole grains and calcium.

Heavy periods

While many people who menstruate won't have severe period-related problems, others aren't so lucky. Heavy periods (medically known as menorrhagia) can massively impact your quality of life, and should not have to be endured. Fear of leakages can deter many women from attending school or work, and prevent them participating in the things they enjoy, like sport or socializing.

I always treat this condition with the utmost seriousness. I often refer patients for an ultrasound scan, which may ascertain why they're bleeding so heavily, and can check for conditions like fibroids, endometriosis, adenomyosis and polycystic ovary syndrome (all of these issues are covered in the second book of this series, *The Power of Female Health, Fertility & Pregnancy*). Once the cause has been pinpointed the bleeding can be managed with tablets such as tranexamic acid or mefenamic acid (the latter tends to be prescribed if you have associated pain, too).

Then, if my patient isn't planning to get pregnant, I can prescribe the combined contraceptive pill or the progesterone-only pill, also known as the mini-pill (see pages 135–8). If that's not suitable, other options include a contraceptive implant or injection (see pages 138–40) or the IUS coil (see page 142). If you've never had a baby, the Jaydess™ or Kyleena™ progesterone-only coil (or 'mini coil') may be prescribed. In extremely severe cases, a patient may be referred to a specialist gynaecologist to discuss the possibility of a hysterectomy (removal of the uterus).

> *If you are using a new pad or tampon hourly or more, then don't suffer in silence. We shouldn't normalize heavy bleeding and your doctor may be able to help.*

Anaemia & periods

Anaemia is a condition characterized by low levels of haemoglobin (iron) in the red blood cells that make up blood. Red blood cells carry oxygen, ferratin, folate and vitamin B12 around your body from your lungs, so they're vital for all bodily functions. Your bone marrow constantly needs iron to make new blood cells to replace older ones that have become worn out or have been lost due to bleeding. However, with frequent bleeding, your body runs low on iron and can't quite keep up in making enough new red blood cells to maintain normal functions. This can lead to the following symptoms:

- Shortness of breath (especially when exercising)
- Palpitations (heart racing)
- Feeling faint
- Looking pale
- Tiredness

A low intake of iron can contribute to anaemia; this can stem from a vegan or vegetarian diet, for example, or from undiagnosed coeliac disease (poor iron absorption is a feature of the latter). Anaemia can also be caused by periods – especially if they're heavy – and affects approximately ten per cent of menstruating women. So, if you have symptoms that are suggestive of anaemia, please make an appointment to see your doctor. They'll assess you fully before performing a simple blood test to measure your blood count and check for coeliac disease. If you are indeed diagnosed with anaemia, this can be corrected by prescribed iron tablets which allow your body to produce enough red blood cells. If you have heavy periods but have not been diagnosed with anaemia or any of the conditions mentioned on page 112, then an over-the-counter supplement of 17–20mg a day, or 210–300mg three times a week, could help.

29% of women of reproductive age are affected by anaemia

Other period-related issues

It's worth talking to a doctor if any of the issues discussed apply to you. Again – and I can't stress this enough – please consider keeping a diary or downloading a tracker app as this will really improve the quality of the consultation with a healthcare professional.

Always seek help if you're worried about your menstrual health.

Puberty & periods: What symptoms might warrant a visit to your doctor?

Puberty and periods are a natural part of growing up, but be aware that sometimes you will need more medical advice. In particular, if you:

- Have started a period before age eight.
- Have not yet had a period and you're aged 16 or above.
- Haven't yet had a period but developed breasts more than three years ago.
- Haven't had any further periods for two years since your first period.
- Are not menstruating regularly every three to six weeks.
- Have missed three periods in a row, or gone 90 days without a period.
- Have extremely heavy bleeding – sometimes called flooding – that soaks through a pad or a tampon (especially if it has to be changed more frequently than every four hours).
- Frequently pass large blood clots (larger than 2.5cm).
- Have periods that last between seven and ten days, as a regular occurrence.
- Have severe PMS/PMDD symptoms (see pages 106–111).
- Have severe cramps that aren't improved by taking simple pain relief, such as paracetamol or ibuprofen.

All women, regardless of age, should also seek medical advice if they experience any vaginal bleeding that seems out of the ordinary, such as:

- Between periods.
- After sex.
- After the menopause (if bleeding restarts after one year of no periods).
- If it's heavier and more painful than usual, especially if you also have symptoms of anaemia (tiredness, looking pale, feeling faint, palpitations/heart racing, shortness of breath – particularly during exercise).

Abnormal bleeding can be a key symptom of three gynaecological cancers (uterine, cervical and vaginal) and is a less common symptom of ovarian cancer. It may also be an indicator of other conditions like endometriosis, adenomyosis, polycystic ovary syndrome (PCOS) and fibroids. In girls and young women, it's commonly understood that the risk of cancer is lower – but if you have any concerns at all, don't hesitate to seek medical advice.

VIOLENCE AGAINST WOMEN & GIRLS

The United Nations defines violence against women and girls (VAWG) as 'gender-based violence that results in, or is likely to result in, physical, sexual or psychological harm or suffering to women, including threats of such acts, coercion or arbitrary deprivation of liberty, whether occurring in public or in private life'.

It's a sad fact that most clinicians, including myself, have encountered patients across the spectrum of age and gender who have experienced abuse or violence. Doctors are trained to recognize the signs (the person may well see the surgery as a 'safe space') and will treat these individuals with the utmost care and sensitivity. Referrals to specialist clinics, services and relevant authorities may occur; these 'multi-agency' approaches are often the most effective way to address the issue.

In an ideal world, human relationships would be positive and pleasurable experiences, free from any coercion, discrimination or violence. Sexual intercourse should only happen in a consensual situation, one in which you feel totally happy and comfortable. You must not feel pressured or threatened to do anything against your will, and you have every right to say no, to exit a situation and to seek a place of refuge.

If you are a victim of any physical, psychological or sexual abuse – including sex trafficking, so-called 'honour' abuse, or intimate image abuse (also known as revenge porn) – please ask for help. You can reach out to a trusted friend or family member, your doctor, a police officer, or a charity helpline or website. I appreciate that stepping forward and speaking up is easier said than done, but rest assured there's a great deal of advice and support available (see Resources on page 187).

Female genital mutilation

Female genital mutilation (FGM) is an abhorrent practice involving the ritualistic cutting of a girl's genitalia (usually her clitoris and/or labia) for 'cultural', non-medical reasons. The practice was outlawed in the UK in 1985, but FGM still takes place around the world. Globally millions of girls remain at risk, most of them of school age.

The physical, mental, sexual and emotional ramifications of FGM are manifold, and include chronic pain, repeated infections and post-traumatic stress disorder (PTSD). The practice can have chronic implications to a woman's wellbeing, and even result in death. Safeguarding patients will always be of paramount importance to doctors, so if an affected individual presents themselves to a surgery we offer them care and attention before organizing referrals to the appropriate medical and/or social services. If the patient is under 18 it is also our legal obligation to inform the police. If you, or someone else, is at risk please seek help.

FGM is child abuse, pure and simple, and it has no place in today's society. Help, advice and support is available from a number of charitable organizations (see Resources on page 188).

CARING FOR YOUR VULVA & VAGINA

Just like the rest of your body, your genitals need lots of TLC and it's vitally important that you keep that area healthy in order to avoid fungal and bacterial infections. You should also be aware of your vaginal discharge in order to spot when something is amiss.

The following is a list of personal hygiene recommendations to help keep your vulva and vagina healthy:

- **Wash your genitals** with clear water and mild, plain soap. Your vulva does not need to smell of flowers. Soap and water are all you need, trust me.
- **Avoid perfumed soaps, gels and oils,** and don't even think about using bath bombs . . . they should be banned in my opinion! Many highly fragranced products use an alcohol base that can make skin dry and sensitive. This in turn disrupts candida in the vulva and can lead to yeast infections and UTIs (urinary tract infections).
- **Shower** instead of having a bath, to avoid scented bath products around the vulval area.
- **Don't use fragranced wipes** as they can upset the healthy balance of pH and bacteria inside the vagina.
- **Don't use abrasive, fragranced toilet tissue,** and rinse with clear water if you can.

- **Avoid 'douching'** (a douche is a device that pushes a stream of water into the vagina).
- **Use mild laundry detergent** to wash your underwear.
- **Avoid wearing tight clothing** and skinny jeans (the bane of my life in my surgery!) as they can trigger vulval irritation.
- **Wear cotton underwear** rather than synthetic – so avoid nylon and polyester – and try to avoid thongs.
- **Avoid wearing underwear in bed,** if possible, although this may not be practical during your period.
- **Change your period protection** regularly.
- **Use a barrier method** of contraception (such as condoms).
- **Pass urine after sex** as it flushes away any cross contamination from the perineal rectal area to the vagina and urethra and can help to prevent UTIs.
- **Avoid hot tubs,** they can be a breeding ground for bacteria and viruses.
- **Maintain a healthy weight** through a nutritious diet and regular exercise.
- **Get to know the triggers** – such as sexual intercourse or your period – that can result in infections.

I know this will be a hard sell for many readers, but I would like to make a particular plea for you to avoid fragranced bath, shower and cleansing products, including those labelled 'feminine' or 'intimate'. Many contain ingredients that disturb the natural balance of vulval and vaginal bacteria and, in my opinion, do much more harm than good. For decades, beauty industry marketing and advertising campaigns have pushed the narrative that women can only keep themselves fresh by using fragranced products, the implication being that female genitals in their natural state are unclean and unhygienic. This fallacy – all too often perpetuated by misogynistic insults about smelly vaginas – is incredibly unhelpful. Wash with water and plain soap is the advice I give to all my patients with vaginas, and it's the advice I'm giving to you, too. So pass it on . . .

Vaginal discharge

Vaginal discharge is a perfectly normal part of women's health – we all experience it – yet we don't pay nearly enough attention to it. It's one of those hush-hush topics that no one seems to talk about but, surprise, surprise, I have no such qualms! Monitoring your secretions means any noticeable changes can prompt you to raise concerns. The frequency and consistency of discharge can vary quite significantly, but colour and odour are clear indications of vaginal health:

- **Clear, relatively odourless discharge** is normal around pregnancy and ovulation, especially if you have had a coil inserted.
- **Whiteish discharge** is usually healthy, but if it has a lumpy consistency, and is accompanied by a burning sensation or itchiness, it might signify a yeast infection.

- **Yellowy-green discharge** is more than likely the result of an STD (see page 161).
- **Greyish discharge** with a fishy smell is a common indicator of bacterial vaginosis (see page 125).
- **Pink-tinged discharge** suggests cervical bleeding or vaginal irritation.
- **Red and bloody discharge** either normal menstrual flow (if occurring around the time of a period) or, in some cases a cervical infection or detached polyp. See your GP if you are concerned.

Colours of vaginal discharge and what they can mean

Your vaginal discharge provides an indication to the overall health of your vagina. Here are the colours you might notice, and what they signify.

CLEAR
Healthy discharge
Pregnancy
Ovulation
Hormonal fluctuations

WHITE
Healthy discharge
Yeast infection, if lumpy and accompanied by itchiness

CARING FOR YOUR VULVA & VAGINA

YELLOW-GREEN
Sexually transmitted disease

RED
Menstruation
Cervical infection
Cervical polyp

PINK
Cervical bleeding
Vaginal irritation
Implantation bleeding

GREY
Bacterial vaginosis

INFECTIONS OF THE GENITALS & URINARY TRACT

Like any other part of the body, the genitals can become infected and minor infections are common and usually easily treatable. Don't suffer in silence. Visit your doctor or pharmacist if you experience the symptoms of these infections. As the urinary tract is situated so close to the anus in female anatomy, infections of this area can be common.

Genital infections

Bacterial vaginosis and thrush are the most common infections that affect the genital area.

Bacterial vaginosis is a common condition that can affect anyone with a vagina from puberty to menopause, particularly those who are sexually active (although it is not a sexually transmitted disease). It is usually caused by a change in the natural pH balance of the bacteria in the vulva and vagina, and one of the signs to watch out for is a thin, watery white-grey vaginal discharge, which can have a fishy odour. Many women have the condition without any symptoms, but if you do have them, you may want to get hold of an over-the-counter test kit from your pharmacy. Bacterial vaginosis generally doesn't cause itching or soreness, so if you notice this I'd suggest you get checked out for thrush or a sexually transmitted disease (see page 161).

Making certain changes to your daily routine can help the symptoms (see page 119), but if things don't improve, your doctor can prescribe antibiotic tablets, gels or creams. If you have a same-sex partner, or share sex toys with someone, you both might need treating. Bacterial vaginosis can sometimes return three months after treatment and, if you are affected more than twice in a month, a longer course of antibiotics may be required.

Thrush is an infection, not a sexually transmitted disease, and is caused by an overgrowth of the *Candida albicans* yeast in the vulval and vaginal area. It's a very common condition that can occur at any age, and can be triggered by many factors, including stress, damage to the skin or poorly controlled diabetes. Thrush is more likely to affect women around ovulation, after sex, or during pregnancy; I myself have suffered with horrendous thrush during all three of my pregnancies – it made me utterly miserable – so I know exactly how awful it can feel. The classic signs are vulval/vaginal soreness and itching – which can often get worse at night – and, sometimes, a cottage cheese-like discharge.

Effective over-the-counter treatment for thrush – a cream and a pessary – can be obtained from your local pharmacy (you can buy self-tests, too). This treatment is effective, but it can take one to two weeks to work properly. If you are having unprotected sex with a male partner, it's wise for him to get treated too; men can carry the yeast, sometimes without symptoms, and can re-infect their partner during sex. He will need to apply the cream onto his penis and foreskin.

Urinary tract infections

Urinary tract infections (UTIs) are incredibly common among girls and women because the urogenital anatomy is in close proximity to the anal area. This means that cross contamination of bugs from the back passage – *E. coli* that lives in the bowel, for example – can easily be transmitted to the bladder, kidneys or urethra (the tube through which urine leaves the body). Cystitis is the name given to inflammation of the bladder, either due to an infectious or non-infectious cause. If bacteria travel up to the kidneys, a condition called pyelonephritis (kidney infection) may be triggered.

UTIs can be painful and distressing but the sooner you recognize the following signs and symptoms, the quicker you'll get treated:

- Burning, stinging or pain when passing urine
- Passing urine more frequently
- Passing small amounts of urine
- Passing more urine than usual during the night
- Irritation to the urethra
- Lower abdominal pain
- Lower back pain
- Raised temperature, fever and/or shivers
- Confusion and disorientation
- Nausea and/or vomiting

My advice is to keep track of your symptoms, drink plenty of water, take paracetamol (a maximum of two

500-milligram tablets, every four to six hours, no more than four times a day) or ibuprofen if tolerated (two 200-milligram tablets, three times a day with food), and use a cold pack on your abdomen to help with the pain. For cystitis, you can buy an over-the-counter treatment in the form of sachets of crystals that are diluted in water; some people find that drinking cranberry juice relieves their symptoms, too.

If you feel you need medical intervention, contact your healthcare provider; if you're given an appointment you'll probably be asked to collect a urine sample, which will be sent to a laboratory to check for bacteria. Your doctor may then prescribe antibiotics to treat the UTI as quickly as possible, although we prefer to be in possession of your results before we do so.

How to prevent UTIs
Recurrent UTIs are common, but the following advice may help prevent them:

- **Always wipe yourself** from front to back (from urethra to anus) after you've been to the toilet.
- **Only use plain soap and clear water** to wash your genitals, and avoid fragranced products.
- **Consider avoiding jacuzzis,** hot tubs and baths, as they can increase the risk of UTIs.
- **Pass urine immediately after sexual intercourse** to clear out your urinary tract.

INFECTIONS OF THE GENITALS & URINARY TRACT

- **Take D-mannose** (a sugar available to buy as a powder or a tablet) every day. It is widely available in health food shops.
- **Drink cranberry juice** every day.
- **Consume probiotics** (lactobacillus), such as sauerkraut, kefir or probiotic yoghurts every day. These contain good bacteria that help the immune system, support gut health and help the body fight off infections, including UTIs.
- **Take topical vaginal oestrogen** if you are perimenopausal or postmenopausal, and are getting recurrent UTIs due to vaginal atrophy (see page 187).
- **Prescribed prophylactic (preventative) antibiotics** from your doctor can stop the infections.

SEXUAL HEALTH & CONTRACEPTION

Firstly, remember that sexual health and contraception are two different elements to consider when you are sexually active. Although there is a lot of crossover between the two, contraception is to prevent pregnancy, while good sexual health practices should reduce your chances of contracting a sexually transmitted infection.

Maintaining good sexual health, and practising safe sex, is a fundamental part of a person's wellbeing. It's a perfectly natural element of everyday life that needs to be discussed honestly and openly without any shame or embarrassment. Previous generations may well have skirted around the subject – talking in riddles about the birds and the bees and the stork that delivers babies – but time has moved on, thank goodness. Nowadays everyone should have the confidence to speak freely and frankly about penises, vaginas, intercourse and condoms.

By having an honest conversation about sex and contraception – with your doctor, school nurse, sexual health practitioner, or relatives you feel comfortable with – you're being extremely sensible and responsible to yourself and any partners that you may have. If you're forearmed and forewarned you'll be less likely to contract (and pass on) harmful sexually transmitted diseases (STDs), and will be more aware of reproductive issues and contraception options (or 'family planning' as it's commonly known).

If you're thinking about engaging in sexual activity for the first time, please be sure in your mind that you feel emotionally and physically ready. If that's the case – and you're not planning to get pregnant – you'll need to research the contraception options available to you. This important fact-finding mission can take the form of a discussion with your doctor or a sexual health nurse, preferably with your partner in tow (it takes two to tango, as they say!). You can also obtain useful information from other trustworthy sources. I always advise my patients to come to their appointment armed with notes and research, since it helps them to make an informed choice, and helps me to tailor their options. It also allows them to make the most of their ten-minute slot, which can pass by very quickly. Reading the next few pages of this book may be helpful to you, I hope, but there is a wealth of information available online (see Resources on page 188).

> Be aware that human papillomavirus can be contracted through oral sex so you should use a dental dam contraception if you are practising oral sex on a vulva with a new partner.

If you're under the age of 16 you are able to visit the doctor alone – this applies to any medical appointment, if that's what you prefer – but in these circumstances your doctor will carefully consider whether you, as a minor, have the ability to make your own independent decisions without parental consent or involvement. The healthcare professional will apply what's called the Gillick competence and Fraser guidelines (see Resources on page 189) to decide this.

A good doctor will adopt a sensitive and non-judgemental approach when discussing contraception and sexual health with all their patients, whatever their age, gender, sexuality or background. Everybody's needs and preferences will differ – individuals belonging to certain faiths and cultures may hold particular views on contraception and family planning, for example – and that should always be respected.

27% of couples practising the withdrawal method will get pregnant each year

Hormonal contraception

If you choose a hormonal method of contraception (either the combined pill, progesterone-only pill, contraceptive injection or implant, or the IUS coil) then it's important to consider that there may be some side effects in the initial stages as your body adjusts. In the vast majority of cases any side effects are minor. Some, such as lighter periods, reduced acne, reduced PMS, may be positive. However, you should keep track of any new symptoms you experience.

These may include:

- Fatigue
- Nausea
- Indigestion

- Constipation
- Difficulty passing urine
- Pain during sexual intercourse
- Bleeding after sexual intercourse
- Weight gain
- Mood changes

Don't hesitate to see your doctor if you need further advice and reassurance.

A note on the withdrawal method & emergency contraception

I will also discuss some methods – the withdrawal method and emergency contraception – that aren't long-term contraceptives but that can lessen chances of pregnancy (see pages 153 and 154), which I know many couples do practise. However, you need to be clear about the failure rates of these types of practices to prevent pregnancy, which are much higher than those when preventative contraception is used.

Which contraceptive products should you choose?

Contraceptives include hormonal options (that prevent your body preparing for pregnancy), barrier methods (that prevent sperm from touching your vagina), or longer-term medical procedures. On the following pages I have described all the main options and how they work.

The combined contraceptive pill
✓ Can reduce heavy periods and cramps
✓ Over 99% effective in preventing pregnancy if taken correctly
✗ Does not provide protection against STDs

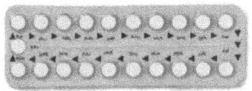

There are many brands, but all contain two hormones – oestrogen and progesterone – and work by stopping the ovaries releasing an egg each month. The usual routine sees women taking one tablet each day for three weeks, and then not taking any for one week of each cycle. The packaging comes labelled with the days of the week for ease of use. In some cases, this regime can be adjusted by your doctor or sexual health nurse to help with period control, period pain and period flow. You may be able to take the Pill continuously for three months, for example, then have a four-day break.

Pros
The combined oral pill is very effective at preventing pregnancy. It regulates menstrual cycles – it often makes them lighter – and can also decrease period cramps. For those who experience heavy menstrual flow, the Pill can help to prevent iron deficiency anaemia (low red blood cell levels). It's also thought to reduce the likelihood of ovarian and uterine cancer, ovarian cysts and pelvic inflammatory disease. Certain types can also be used as a treatment for acne.

Cons
You need to take a tablet at the same time every day (I advise patients to put a reminder on their phone), and its effectiveness can be reduced if you suffer with prolonged vomiting and/or diarrhoea. It can't be used by everyone – it may not be prescribed to women who are obese or who smoke heavily, for example – and possible side effects can include nausea, headaches, strokes and blood clots. The Pill can also affect your libido, your mood and cause weight gain. It doesn't protect against STDs either, so you'll still need to use a condom if you have multiple partners or a new partner.

SEXUAL HEALTH & CONTRACEPTION

The progesterone-only pill
✓ Can reduce heavy periods and cramps
✓ Over 99% effective in preventing pregnancy if taken correctly
✗ Must be taken at the same time each day
✗ Does not provide protection against STDs

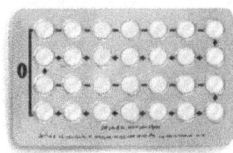

The progesterone-only pill (POP), also known as the mini-pill, is available over the counter under various brand names. The POP contains only one hormone, progesterone, and works by thickening the cervical mucus and preventing the sperm reaching the egg. The packaging comes labelled with the days of the week for ease of use.

There's a strict time window in which the POP must be taken each day if you are having unprotected sex. There are essentially two groups of POP:

Group 1 must be taken within 12 hours of the same time each day.

Group 2, the traditional POP, must be taken within three hours of the same time each day.

Pros

The POP shares similar advantages with the combined contraceptive pill (see page 135) but, since it only has one hormone, it offers less of a risk regarding clots and migraines. Some mini-pills may help with period cramps and PMS (your doctor will tell you more) and it is also safe to take while breastfeeding. Some brands (containing norethindrone acetate or dienogest) are used to treat endometriosis symptoms. If taken correctly, it is more than 99 per cent effective.

Cons

You need to take a tablet at the same time every day (I advise patients to put a reminder on their phone), and its effectiveness can be reduced if you suffer with prolonged vomiting and/or diarrhoea. Side effects from this medication may include acne, nausea, lower libido, mood swings, breast tenderness/swelling and increased vaginal discharge. In some patients with hypermobility, progesterone-only contraception can make their symptoms, such as joint pain, worse. As with the combined pill, it will not protect you against STDs so you'll need to use a condom if you have multiple partners or a new partner.

The contraceptive implant

✓ Over 99% effective in preventing pregnancy
✓ Can cause fewer or lighter periods
✓ Once inserted, it lasts for three years so you don't need to remember to take a tablet
✓ A good option for women who can't use oestrogen-based contraception
✗ Does not provide protection against STDs

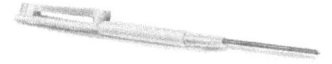

The implant is a small, bendy plastic rod that a doctor or nurse inserts beneath the skin of your upper arm. It lasts for three years, and stops you from getting pregnant by releasing progesterone into the bloodstream.

Pros
The implant is over 99 per cent effective, so it protects you very well against pregnancy. As it's a long-term contraceptive, you won't have to think about it for another three years (and you won't have to worry about forgetting a pill). It's a good option for women who can't use contraception that contains

oestrogen, and it may also cause fewer or lighter menstrual periods.

Cons
Insertion involves minor surgery, which is off-putting to some, and there's a small risk of infection following the procedure. The implant may give you side effects that can include acne, depression, hair loss, weight gain and disrupted menstrual periods. It doesn't protect against STDs either, so you'll still need to use a condom if you have multiple partners or a new partner.

Contraceptive injection

- ✓ 99% effective in preventing pregnancy
- ✓ Lasts for three months so you don't need to remember to take a tablet
- ✓ A good option for women who can't use oestrogen-based contraception
- ✗ Does not provide protection against STDs

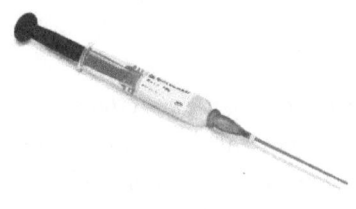

The contraceptive injection is administered by a healthcare professional. Each injection contains a dose of progesterone and provides three months of protection against pregnancy. It works by thinning the lining of the endometrium and increasing the thickness of the cervical mucus, therefore not allowing sperm to reach the egg, so avoiding fertilization and implantation.

Pros
The injection is an excellent contraceptive method (it's 99 per cent effective) and is suitable for those who can't be given oestrogen, as well as those who might worry about forgetting to take a tablet every day. Some women may stop getting menstrual periods, which may come as a relief, and studies have shown that it can help to protect against uterine cancer. As with the Pill, coil and implant, it doesn't interrupt sexual activity.

Cons
Reported side effects have included tiredness and weight gain. Some studies have shown that continuous use of the contraceptive injection for more than two years can lead to bone density loss, therefore an annual review and assessment by your doctor is necessary; they may recommend an alternative method of contraception if you have risk factors such as having anorexia nervosa (an eating disorder) or being on corticosteroid therapy (for autoimmune conditions, or rheumatoid arthritis, for example).

Some women may have irregular menstrual bleeding or spotting for up to six months after the injection, occasionally for even longer. In some patients with hypermobility, progesterone-only contraception can make their symptoms, such as joint pain, worse. You need to make a note to visit the doctor every three months to get the injection topped up. It doesn't protect against STDs so you'll still need to use a condom if you have multiple partners or a new partner.

The IUS coil

✓ Over 99% effective in preventing pregnancy
✓ Inserted by a healthcare professional so you don't have to worry about remembering it
✗ Does not provide protection against STDs

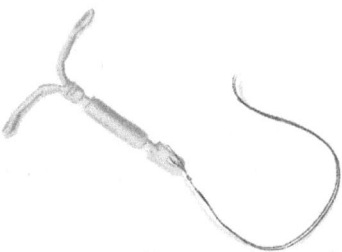

The IUS (intra-uterine system) coil is a hormone-releasing, small, T-shaped implement inserted into the uterus. It releases small amounts of progesterone into the uterus, which alters the cervical mucus and makes it difficult for sperm to survive and reach the egg. It sometimes stops ovulation and helps to reduce blood flow to the endometrium, so periods can be less heavy and painful.

Pros

The IUS coil is extremely effective, it only has a 0.2 per cent failure rate each year. A mini progesterone coil is also available that might be more comfortable for some people. Once inserted, the IUS can be kept in for five years, providing long-term protection without needing daily attention or regular checks. It's comfortable – neither you nor your partner will feel it's there – and some women find it lessens (or even stops) menstrual flow and prevents worsening of endometriosis. The IUS can also prevent fluctuations in hormones, which can improve symptoms of PMS and PMDD. This particular coil may also be a good option for women who have previously suffered blood clots, pulmonary embolism (PE) or deep vein thrombosis (DVT). The Mirena™ IUS coil can also be used as the progesterone component of hormone replacement therapy for five years.

Cons

The procedure can be painful, but it only takes five to ten minutes, and there are a number of pain relief methods that can be used, such as taking paracetamol and ibuprofen an hour before the procedure, your doctor applying a local anaesthetic gel when inserting the speculum and apply a 10 per cent lidocaine spray to the cervix. In some cases, a cervical block (a local anaesthetic injection) can be administered.

There is a slight risk of infection in the first 20 days after insertion, and there's a small chance (0.5–0.8 per cent) of it falling out (the risk varies, but it is slightly higher in 14–19-year-olds or for patients with Ehlers-Danlos Syndrome/hypermobility). There is an even smaller risk of it puncturing the uterus. In some patients with hypermobility, progesterone-only contraception can make their symptoms worse. It doesn't protect against STDs so you'll need to use a condom if you have multiple partners or a new partner.

The Vaginal Ring

- ✓ Over 99% effective in preventing pregnancy if used correctly
- ✓ Self-inserted once a month so you don't have to worry about remembering it daily
- ✗ Does not provide protection against STDs

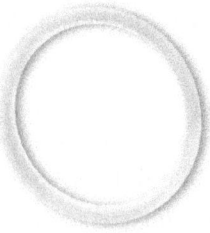

The vaginal ring, sometimes referred to as a NuvaRing™, is a soft plastic ring that releases a continuous dose of oestrogen and progestogen. This works in the same way as the combined contraceptive pill to prevent pregnancy by stopping the ovaries from releasing an egg each month. It is inserted into the vagina with your fingers and should then be kept in place for 21 days. After 21 days it is removed from the vagina and left out for 7 days, which will lead to a monthly bleed. After 7 days a new ring should be inserted and the cycle continues.

Pros

If used correctly, the vaginal ring is extremely effective in preventing pregnancy, and if you insert it within 5 days of the start of your period, it will be effective straight away. It is suitable for people who are confident they will remember the routine of when to insert and remove it but don't want to remember to take a daily pill. As with other hormonal options, it can make periods lighter and less painful, and reduce PMS symptoms. If you would prefer not to have a monthly bleed then you can insert a new ring straight after removing the old one, or have a shorter break (than 7 days) between rings.

Cons

You need to remember when to insert it and when to remove it each month. If you start using it more than 5 days after the start of your period you will also need to use additional contraception until the ring has been inserted for 7 days. It can't be used by everyone – it may not be prescribed to women who are overweight or who smoke, for example – and possible side effects can include nausea, headaches, strokes and blood clots. Some people and their partners can feel the ring during sex, this does not mean it is inserted incorrectly, however. Occasionally the ring can come out on its own. If this happens you should re-insert the ring (if it happens in the first week) or insert a new ring (if it happens in week two or three) and use additional contraception for 7 days. Prescriptions are usually available as a batch of 4 months' worth so you will need fairly regular trips to your doctor or sexual health clinic to renew the prescription. It doesn't protect against STDs so you'll need to use a condom if you have multiple partners or a new partner.

The IUD coil

- ✓ Over 99% effective in preventing pregnancy
- ✓ Inserted by a healthcare professional so you don't have to worry about remembering it or taking it correctly
- ✓ A good option for women who want very reliable contraception without taking hormones
- ✗ Does not provide protection against STDs

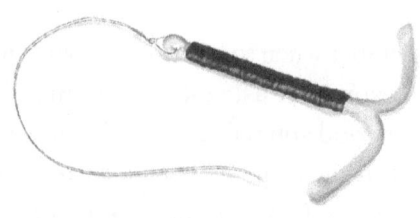

The IUD (intra-uterine device) coil is a small, T-shaped implement that is inserted into the uterus. It does not contain any hormones but releases a small amount of copper into the uterus, which weakens sperm and stops it from reaching an egg.

Pros

The IUD coil is extremely effective in preventing pregnancy, it has only a 0.1 per cent failure rate each year. Once inserted, it can remain in place for ten years so provides long-term protection and doesn't require daily attention or regular checks; you just leave it in situ. It's comfortable – neither you nor your partner will feel it's there – and is a great option for women who've had breast cancer and need to avoid hormones.

Cons

As with the IUS coil, the procedure can be painful, but it takes only five to ten minutes, and there are a number of pain relief methods that can be used, such as taking paracetamol and ibuprofen an hour before the procedure, your doctor applying a local anaesthetic gel when inserting the speculum and applying a 10 per cent lidocaine spray to the cervix. In some cases, a cervical block (a local anaesthetic injection) can be administered, but for some women the needle can cause pain.

There is a slight risk of infection in the first 20 days after coil insertion, and there's a small chance (0.5–0.8 per cent) of it falling out (the risk varies, but studies have shown it is slightly higher in 14–19-year-olds, in patients with Ehlers-Danlos Syndrome, a connective tissue disorder, and if it's inserted immediately after a vaginal birth). There is an even smaller risk of a coil puncturing the uterus. The copper coil can have some side effects, including longer and heavier periods, increased cramping and occasional spotting. It doesn't protect against STDs so you'll need to use a condom if you have multiple partners or a new partner.

Male condoms

✓ Offers significant protection against STDs if used correctly

✓ Widely available without needing access to a healthcare professional

✓ 98% effective in preventing pregnancy if used correctly

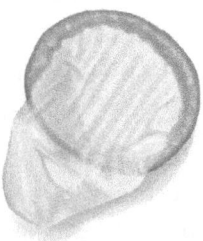

A condom is a thin sheath, usually made of latex, that is rolled over a penis before sexual intercourse. It works as a barrier to stop semen from touching the vagina. Remember that with all male condoms, withdrawal should happen soon after ejaculation to avoid sperm leaking into the vagina.

Pros

If used correctly, condoms are 98 per cent effective in preventing pregnancy. They also significantly reduce your risk (and your partner's risk) of contracting sexually transmitted diseases. They are widely available to purchase from pharmacies, supermarkets and garages (as well as many bars and restaurants) and can sometimes be obtained free of charge from sexual health centres. They also enable men to play an active part in preventing pregnancy (instead of the onus being on the woman) and, since they don't require advance preparation, are an ideal way to protect yourself during unplanned sexual encounters. In most cases, condoms have no medical side effects.

Cons

You have to use a new condom each time you have intercourse and, because they're not generally available on prescription, this can be expensive. Having to put it on the penis before penetration means that sexual activity can be disrupted, although many couples happily incorporate it into their foreplay. There's a risk that the condom will tear or slip off during sex, so it's not the most failsafe method of contraception.

Condoms made from latex are unsuitable for anyone who's allergic to latex, but other materials are available: polyisoprene condoms, which are made from synthetic rubber that is stretchy and provides a good fit; or polyurethane condoms, which are made from plastic rather than latex, so don't always fit very snugly and can slip off.

Lambskin, or 'natural', condoms made from sheep intestines are also available. These work to prevent pregnancy but do not protect against STDs because the material is porous and allows tiny viruses to get through.

Female condoms

✓ Offers good protection against STDs if used correctly
✓ Can be inserted long before sexual intercourse
✓ 95% effective in preventing pregnancy if used properly

Worn inside the woman's vagina, the female condom is made from thin latex and works by creating a barrier to prevent sperm reaching the uterus.

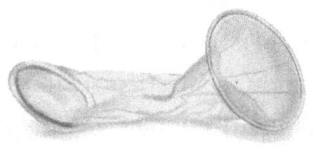

Pros
Female condoms are available to buy from some pharmacies (and can be obtained from sexual health clinics) and, if used correctly, can offer good protection against STDs. Unlike the male version, the female condom can be inserted long before intercourse (so there's less interruption to sexual

activity) and the man does not need to withdraw his penis immediately after ejaculation. There are no medical side effects, other than triggering allergic reactions to latex.

Cons
Mastering the insertion technique can be tricky for many women, and the condom may feel a little uncomfortable when inside the vagina. If female condoms are used properly, they are 95 per cent effective, so are less reliable than other contraceptive methods. You need to use a new condom each time you have intercourse and, unlike the male version, they are not always widely available to buy on the high street. Female condoms made from latex are unsuitable for anyone who's allergic to latex.

Diaphragm

- ✓ Can be inserted up to two hours before sexual intercourse
- ✓ More environmentally friendly because it can be re-used for two years
- ✓ 92% effective in preventing pregnancy if used properly with spermicide
- ✗ Does not offer reliable protection against STDs

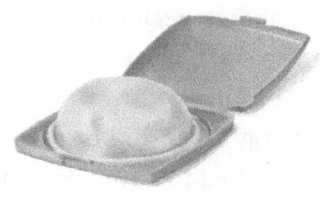

The diaphragm, also known as the cap, is a barrier method of contraception which is inserted into the vagina to fit over the cervix before sexual intercourse. It's usually used with spermicidal gel. There are different sizes available and you would usually be fitted for one by a healthcare professional (although there is now a one-size-fits-all diaphragm that can be purchased online, too). It needs to stay in place for at least six hours after sexual intercourse to be effective.

Pros
Being a barrier method of contraception, it contains no hormones and will have no physical impact on your body (such as period disruption, breast tenderness, mood changes or low libido). The diaphragm gives the woman full control – it can be inserted up to two hours before sex – and, when washed after each use, one diaphragm can last for two years. Being so long-lasting means it is the most environmentally friendly barrier method.

Cons
This barrier method is not as effective as others. The one-size-fits-all diaphragm may be even less effective than a fitted diaphragm, with studies showing that, with *typical* use, 17 out of 100 women will become pregnant after one year. Getting the diaphragm technique right can be tricky and fiddly; before you start using it, you'll need to make an appointment for a fitting with your doctor or nurse to double-check it's the right size and being put in the right place. You may need to be fitted for a new diaphragm (or

cap) if you lose or gain more than 3kg in weight or have an abortion, and you should always be fitted for a new diaphragm after you have given birth.

Female sterilization

✓ Permanent, non-reversible option for people who do not want to ever be pregnant
✗ Does not provide protection against STDs

A tubal ligation is a minor surgical procedure that cuts or blocks the fallopian tubes. A hysterectomy is a more serious operation which removes the uterus (often carried out to treat conditions like uterine fibroids and pelvic pain). Both of these procedures are performed by a gynaecologist.

Pros
Both procedures are highly effective against pregnancy, since they offer permanent protection. They are options for someone who is certain they don't want to get pregnant, or does not want to have any more children. A hysterectomy will stop your periods, and will remove any risk of uterine or cervical cancer.

Cons
Tubal ligation may involve some pain. It does not affect your menstrual cycles and does not prevent any gynaecological cancers. A hysterectomy can have a very long recovery time. Both surgeries are non-reversible, and don't protect against STDs so you'll need to use a condom if you have multiple partners or a new partner.

Withdrawal technique
✗ Not a reliable contraceptive option
✗ Does not provide protection against STDs
✓ 73% effective in preventing pregnancy

The withdrawal technique relies on a man withdrawing his penis from a woman's vagina before ejaculation. It is not a reliable contraceptive option but is sometimes used alongside period tracking to lessen the chance of pregnancy.

Pros
This is a natural, non-medical method with no cost implications. There are no physical or medical side effects, and it allows a man to play an active part in pregnancy prevention.

Cons
The withdrawal technique is not an effective method of contraception, primarily because it is difficult for a man to predict ejaculation, and the penis can leak some sperm in the prostatic fluid (pre-cum) before ejaculation. It has only a 73 per cent success rate, which means 27 out of 100 women using this withdrawal method for a year will become unintentionally pregnant. The associated worry about getting pregnant can decrease sexual pleasure for both parties

and, without a barrier such as a condom, it doesn't protect against STDs.

Emergency contraception

✓ The morning-after pill is at least 97% effective at preventing pregnancy if used properly (varies between brands)

✓ The IUD coil is over 99.9% effective at preventing pregnancy if fitted within five days of unprotected sex

✗ Does not provide protection against STDs

✗ Emergency contraception should not be used as your regular method

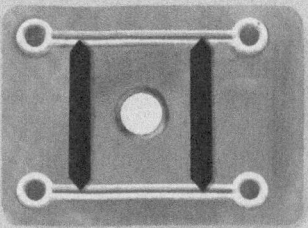

These are birth-control measures taken after you've had unprotected sex, in order to prevent pregnancy. The morning-after pill works by preventing or delaying ovulation and, in order to maximize effectiveness, should be taken as soon as possible after unprotected sex. The morning-after pill is available over the counter from most pharmacies, and does not require a prescription. Under current plans it will be free of charge from pharmacies nationwide from late 2025 onwards. Some brands have to be taken within 72 hours (3 days) of sex, and others have to be taken within 120 hours (5 days) of sex. The IUD coil (see page 146) stops an egg from being fertilized or implanting in the uterus, and can be inserted into the uterus as an emergency intervention up to five days after unprotected sex, or up to five days after the earliest time the person could have ovulated.

Pros
These methods are very effective at preventing pregnancy and you'll have a less than 0.1% chance of getting pregnant if the IUD coil is fitted within five days of unprotected sex, and a 3% chance if the morning-after pill is taken as directed.

Cons
Morning-after pills are not effective if you vomit within three hours of taking them, so you may need another dose. They can also cause bloating, nausea and breast tenderness, and could make your menstrual cycle irregular. The IUD coil will need to be inserted at your doctor's surgery, and can be painful (see page 146). Neither of these methods protect against sexually transmitted diseases.

UNPLANNED PREGNANCY

If you are having intercourse, there is always a chance that you will become pregnant. Pregnancy tests are available over the counter in pharmacies and can be taken from the first day of a missed period. Before you confirm things with a test, you may already have a suspicion you are pregnant. A missed menstrual period is the most obvious sign, but other tell-tale symptoms can include tender, swollen breasts, a change in mood, and nausea (with or without vomiting). A pregnancy test is simple to take and involves weeing on a stick and then waiting a few minutes for the result to show on the stick (follow the instructions provided with the test).

If the result is positive, and you were not planning on having a baby at this time, you may feel lots of different emotions. Firstly, try not to panic; unexpected pregnancies can happen to any of us. Once you've got over the shock you will, of course, have to assess your options and decide how you wish to proceed. In order to help you with this, I'd urge you to talk things through with your partner, or a trusted friend or family member, someone well placed to give you sensible, rational advice. But if you feel you can't talk to a loved one, you can book an appointment with your doctor or practice nurse, either of whom will treat you with care and sensitivity and will offer you informed and non-judgemental advice. There is also a wealth of advice available from charities and other organizations, too (see Resources on page 188). Essentially, your options are:

- Continuing with the pregnancy and raising the baby yourself or with your family
- Having an abortion to terminate the pregnancy
- Continuing with the pregnancy and having the baby adopted

Continuing with a pregnancy

Should you decide to go ahead with the pregnancy, then make an appointment with your GP (sometimes called a 'booking in' appointment). Here, you'll receive all the necessary antenatal advice, will be referred to your local hospital's maternity services, and will be listed for all the requisite scans and screenings. You might also like to find a copy of the second book in my series – *The Power of Female Health, Fertility & Pregnancy* – to get an idea of what to expect during pregnancy and childbirth. If you choose to continue with the pregnancy and have your baby adopted after the birth, this process would ordinarily be looked after by a local authority's social services department and/or an adoption agency.

Ending a pregnancy

If you live in England, Wales or Scotland and decide to terminate the pregnancy before 24 weeks, please make an appointment as soon as possible with your doctor, sexual health clinic or the British Pregnancy Advice Service

(BPAS). A clinician will advise you and counsel you, without judgement or prejudice, and will refer you to an abortion clinic for further assessment and treatment. After 24 weeks, a termination can only be performed under extreme circumstances, for example if the mother's life is at risk or the child is likely to be born with severe disability. You may also refer yourself to a private abortion clinic, where you'll have to pay for the procedure (the costs vary). Your local NHS sexual health clinic will have details of nearby services.

If you are under 16, your parents do not need to be told you are planning a termination, but you may be encouraged (but not pressured) to confide in a loved one for physical and mental support. Sometimes a family doctor will refer a patient to another colleague in the surgery if they are unable to participate in abortion for religious or ethical reasons. Ending a pregnancy can be a traumatic experience that necessitates lots of help and support. See Resources on page 188 for organizations that offer advice and guidance.

The abortion law in Northern Ireland changed in March 2020. Women currently have access to a termination up until 12 weeks gestation (that is, 11 weeks and 6 days) without any conditions, and from 12 to 24 weeks if the pregnancy is impacting the woman's physical or mental health. Please consult the NHS website for the most up-to-date guidelines.

SEXUALLY TRANSMITTED DISEASES

Sexually transmitted diseases (also known as STDs or STIs – sexually transmitted infections) are a risk for anyone who has sexual intercourse or sexual contact with other people. It is vital that you know how to protect yourself from contracting them, and that you are aware of the early signs of STDs so that you can seek treatment.

Those who don't use barrier methods of contraception are particularly susceptible to STDs. Note that STDs can occur at any stage in your life, too, and – contrary to popular opinion – are not just restricted to people in their teens, twenties and thirties. I've definitely noticed an increase in older patients presenting with STD symptoms, particularly midlife women who – once their periods cease and their pregnancy risk abates – are choosing not to use condoms.

First and foremost, I'd advise anyone who's having sex to consider using barrier methods of contraception, even if you're on the Pill (and especially if you have a new partner or multiple partners). STDs can cause some really unpleasant symptoms yet can be easily avoided by taking a responsible approach to your own sexual health, and perhaps keeping a few condoms in your bag. It's also a good idea to familiarize yourself with your local sexual health clinic (sometimes called a genitourinary medicine or GUM clinic) should you ever need to visit it. Every area should have one of these specialist centres, which offers a range of confidential and non-judgemental services, including testing and treatment. They are usually accessed by making an appointment or by attending drop-in sessions (some clinics are aimed at specific groups, including young people and LGBTQ+ communities).

You should always book in for an STD screening if you notice any of the tell-tale symptoms, have had unprotected sex, or have shared a needle or suffered an accidental needlestick injury. All STD centres have a secure and confidential contact-tracing system so they'll contact any current or former partners on your behalf.

You can also get any STD symptoms looked at by your doctor, if you prefer. And please don't feel embarrassed at the prospect of a clinician examining your genitals. We are so experienced in this field (I've seen thousands of vulvas and vaginas) and will always treat patients with the utmost care and respect.

> Many STDs can be treated by antibiotics or antivirals, but you can catch them more than once, therefore practising safe sex is vitally important.

These days, it's not uncommon for couples in the early stage of a relationship to get themselves checked out for STDs before they have sex (people in some local authority areas can receive free chlamydia, gonorrhoea and HIV self-testing kits delivered to their door). A trip to the GUM clinic may not be the most romantic date you'll ever go on, but it's one of the most responsible things you can do for each other.

I think it's really important that young people recognize the various STD symptoms. Granted, the following may not necessarily make pleasant reading, but it will help you spot the signs early and avoid future complications.

The herpes virus

There are two types of herpes virus: type 1 herpes causes cold sores on the face, and type 2 causes sores on the genitals. The latter is a common STD that's passed on through sex (vaginal, oral or anal). An outbreak can cause small blisters around the genitals and is usually accompanied by a tingling, burning and itching sensation. These blisters can often burst open, exuding a clear liquid and leaving red open sores (women can also suffer vaginal discharge). The herpes virus can live in your body for years and then reappear, even if you've not had sex. There is no cure for it, but your doctor or STD clinic may be able to prescribe anti-viral medication to stop or reduce the severity of an outbreak.

Chlamydia

This is a very common STD that can easily be passed from person to person because sufferers can be symptom-free; indeed, some women only realize they have the infection years afterwards, when they have difficulty becoming pregnant. Those that do have symptoms often notice an unusual vaginal or penile discharge, pain on passing urine, pain when having sex, or pain in the abdominal area. Some women with chlamydia feel an ache when they're having a period. Chlamydia can be treated with antibiotics.

Gonorrhoea
This is caused by a bacterium that affects men and women. Not everyone will have symptoms, but the key sign is a thick, yellow-green penile or vaginal discharge. Other symptoms include pelvic pain, pain while passing urine or stools, and bleeding during or after sex. Women can suffer bleeding between periods and, although rare, men can experience swollen testicles. Gonorrhoea can be treated with antibiotics.

Trichomoniasis
This is caused by a parasite. It produces a yellow-green vaginal discharge that can be thick, thin or frothy, with a strong, fishy odour. Other signs include genital soreness and itching, and pain while passing urine. Half of trichomoniasis sufferers have no symptoms, so it can be easily passed on. Trichomoniasis can be treated with antibiotics.

Syphilis
This is caused by a bacterium, and symptoms might not always be obvious. They can include fever, fatigue, sore throat, aching joints, white patches in the mouth and swollen lymph nodes. Some people suffer a blotchy rash on the palms of the hands and the soles of the feet. Painless sores or ulcers around the vulva and anus can sometimes go unnoticed. Syphilis can be treated with antibiotics.

Pubic lice

Also known as 'crabs', lice can cause itching around the pubic area. Some sufferers notice small white or pale-bluish spots around the genitals, thighs and lower abdominal area, and others can feel tired and run down. Pubic lice are treated by a malathion or permethrin lotion, which should be applied and left on for 12 hours then washed off. The treatment will need to be repeated seven days later to ensure that all the lice have been eradicated.

Human papillomavirus (HPV)

This is in fact a group of around 100 different viruses, although not all are sexually transmitted. HPV is transmitted by genital skin contact, by vaginal, anal or oral sex, or by sharing sex toys. In most cases, men and women don't realize they have it, although a low-risk HPV may cause genital warts or an oral infection. A high-risk HPV may cause cell changes at the cervix that can cause cancer but this can be spotted and addressed during a routine cervical screening (otherwise known as a smear test). These tests are offered every three years to women aged between 25 and 49, and every five years to women aged between 50 and 64.

In the UK, all boys and girls born on or after 1 September 2006 are offered the HPV vaccine when they are aged between 12 and 13. The vaccine is offered to people up to 45 years old, but it's thought to be most effective when administered to a person before they become sexually active. Statistics in 2022 showed that HPV vaccines provided 87 per cent protection against cervical cancer.

HIV (human immunodeficiency virus)
HIV is a sexually transmitted infection that can damage your immune system. Initial symptoms can be very vague, and can include weight loss, lack of energy, night sweats and recurrent infections. If HIV remains untreated, it can progress to a disease known as acquired immunodeficiency syndrome (AIDS).

HIV still remains a global issue, with no cure for the infection as such. However, thanks to huge advances in medical science, we now live in an age when HIV testing, diagnosis and treatment has become incredibly effective, so much so that the infection can be controlled by medication, and does not necessarily lead to AIDS. This wonderful development means that people with HIV are now able to live long and healthy lives. You can obtain an HIV test from your local sexual health clinic (it's free in some areas of the UK) or via charities such as the excellent Terrence Higgins Trust (see Resources on page 188).

CONSIDERATIONS FOR TRANS INDIVIDUALS

In the following section, I shall largely use 'trans' as an umbrella term, but this refers to anyone with a uterus who defines themselves as transgender, non-binary or gender diverse.

The General Medical Council (GMC) states that 'trans and non-binary people experience the same health problems as everyone else, and have very few differing needs. If a health problem is related to gender identity, or its treatment, you must assess, provide treatment for and refer trans patients the same as you would other patients.'

Sadly, this guidance doesn't always apply in practice. For myriad reasons, many trans and non-binary people continue to suffer medical discrimination across the healthcare spectrum. This is something that needs to change, starting with more allies and advocates within surgeries and hospitals. As a GP, I'm committed to helping and supporting *all* patients, whether they happen to identify as cis gender, trans or otherwise.

Those assigned female at birth (AFAB) who no longer identify with that gender will require healthcare that's within my specialist remit and, like all my patients, will be treated with respect, and without bias. I am very conscious that I am often their first point of contact within a healthcare setting.

Much of the clinical guidance already outlined in this chapter will apply to a trans person who possesses a uterus. For example, I'll offer them the same advice about tracking their menstrual cycles, selecting appropriate contraception and monitoring their sexual health. They may well require treatment for issues such as endometriosis, premenstrual syndrome (PMS) or polycystic ovary syndrome (PCOS). However, I'm acutely aware that some trans people suffer with gender dysphoria, and will always take this into account.

According to the NHS, 'gender dysphoria is a term that describes a sense of unease that a person may have because their gender identity doesn't match their birth sex. This sense of unease or dissatisfaction may be so intense it can lead to depression and anxiety and have a harmful impact on daily life.'

Some trans people are fearful of (or repulsed by) their own anatomical features and characteristics, which can lead to feelings of anxiety and vulnerability during a clinical appointment or an examination. In these situations, I'll always do my very best to ease their worries and make them feel as comfortable as possible, which may include adopting different terminology, ensuring I use their preferred pronouns, or avoiding assumptions about their sexual preferences.

Trans men can present with distinct physiological and emotional needs and issues that may relate to the following areas.

Menstruation

Monthly periods can be deeply problematic for a trans person suffering with dysphoria. If they wish to stop their menstrual cycle, we can discuss the suitability of long-term contraceptives, such as an implant or IUS coil. Younger patients, or perhaps those who've not had children, can be fitted with a more compact coil.

The contraceptive pill is another option. If a patient is not on testosterone therapy then they can be prescribed the combined contraceptive pill, which can be taken continuously for three months with a four-day break, reducing the number of periods they experience. If a patient is on testosterone therapy then they can be prescribed the progesterone-only mini-pill, that can be taken continuously so they do not have periods. However, as the IUS and both contraceptive pills are hormonal treatments, consideration needs to be given to any other hormones a trans person might be prescribed as part of their gender affirmation therapy (such as testosterone).

Fertility

If a trans patient with a uterus decides to embark on hormone treatment, yet still wishes to have biological children in the future, they may consider egg preservation; the Human Fertilisation and Embryology Authority (HFEA) website contains a wealth of information about this (see Resources on page 189).

Local Integrated Care Systems in England, Scotland and Wales should provide funding for fertility for trans patients and their policies should support *all* patients undergoing NHS treatment that is likely to affect their fertility.

Mental health

Trans people are disproportionately affected by mental ill health that can be aggravated by the bigotry and prejudice they often face. Malicious misgendering, for example, or legal and social discrimination can exacerbate poor emotional wellbeing. The *Stonewall LGBT in Britain Health Report*, published in 2018, makes for disturbing reading. Results from a study group of 5,000 people found that 71 per cent of trans individuals had experienced anxiety during the previous year, with 35 per cent admitting to self-harm. Almost half of trans people (46 per cent) had experienced suicidal thoughts and 12 per cent had attempted to end their lives. I'm always mindful of these statistics, and I believe other clinicians should be, too. I really recommend the Stonewall website for further reading (see Resources on page 189).

Eating disorders

Trans people, especially those suffering with dysphoria, can be particularly susceptible to eating disorders such as anorexia or bulimia (the Stonewall Report put the figure at 21 per cent, so that's roughly one in five). Being underweight can prompt the cessation or disruption of menstrual periods, and/or can reduce the size of breasts, which is often the ulterior motive. Doctors like myself need to be aware of this and, if necessary, refer the patient for specialist support.

Your GP will signpost you to the specialist care and treatment you require. Ask the surgery receptionist which doctor is best placed to help you.

Gender identity

At the time of writing, if you live in the UK, are 18 or over and are transgender, you can ask your doctor to refer you to a gender identity clinic, also known as a gender dysphoria clinic or GDC (see Resources on page 188 for more information). There, you'll receive specialist care that can range from psychological help to hormone therapy. With regard to the latter, trans women are typically prescribed oestrogen along with testosterone blockers, whereas trans men usually receive testosterone (and sometimes oestrogen blockers). Your GP will be kept in the loop by the GDC, and will be on hand to offer general practice-based support if you require it.

If you're under the age of 18 and are transgender, your family doctor can refer you to the Gender Identity Development Service (GIDS) that caters for the needs of children and young people. GPs will apply Gillick competence guidelines (see Resources on page 189) to any patient under the age of 16 who does not wish to involve their parents. The multidisciplinary team will offer you a wide range of services and resources, which may involve counselling and hormone therapy. As you approach adulthood, GIDS may refer you on to a Gender Identity Clinic where you can progress towards more permanent gender affirmation treatments. There is some useful information available online (see Resources on page 188).

Chest binding

Chest binders are tight-fitting, elasticated vests that some trans men and non-binary people wear to flatten their breast tissue. The majority of these garments are made to strict specifications in order to meet safety standards, but it's often a good idea for a doctor to double-check that they're fitting properly. Overly tight binders can cause pain to the chest wall and ribs and can prevent sleep due to soreness. They can also cut into the skin, which may cause skin infections such as cellulitis. Even if you bind your chest, be sure to regularly examine the breast tissue for lumps (see pages 19–23).

46% of trans people in the UK have experienced suicidal thoughts

DR NIGHAT'S TAKEAWAYS

1 See the doctor who's right for you
Make sure you register with your local healthcare provider and, if possible, ask to be seen by a clinician who specializes in women's or trans health.

2 Know your body and track your menstrual cycle
Download a period-tracking app onto your phone or note symptoms in a diary; it'll help you understand your monthly cycle (and your doctor will love you for it!).

3 Don't put up with period pain
Don't be a martyr to your pain! Paracetamol (and ibuprofen, if you can take it) can ease your symptoms and help you get on with life.

4 Weigh up your health options
Do your research, and choose the period products and contraceptive methods that best suit you. What's right for one person may not be right for another.

5 Share your views, concerns & expectations
Empower yourself – you're in charge! Outline your worries to your doctor, ask them lots of questions and discuss how your symptoms can be managed.

SHARING THE KNOWLEDGE

Throughout our lives we need to be able to keep checking and understanding our bodies. Know what is normal for you. Understand when something is not right and know when to go to your doctor to show your concern.

I want to emphasize that the stigma and taboo around women's health and women's biology ends with this book. Enough with the lack of diversity and inclusion in medical textbooks. Enough with misrepresentation of neurodiverse women and those who are differently abled. Enough of ignoring ethnic minority communities. Enough of undermining and gaslighting women's bodies and their symptoms. Enough with not providing adequate pain relief for smear tests, childbirth and hysteroscopies. Enough of not showing real-life body shapes. Enough of lack of data. Enough of medical misogyny, which is perpetrated by the patriarchy – including the patriarchy within us and our own misgivings about whether our pain is worth discussing.

Hopefully by now you've recognized that I have absolutely no qualms talking about breasts, vulvas, vaginas, anuses – the lot! I think it's so important for women to be queens of their bodies, and as queens we should be fixing each other's crowns along the way.

This book is not mine; it is my gift to you. Take the

knowledge within this book and share it like confetti with those around you.

Nighat Arif

Dr Nighat Arif

This book is my gift to you: take it, look after it, come back to it when you're ready, and know that you have the freedom to choose the care that suits you.

GLOSSARY OF WOMEN'S HEALTH

Abdomen The region of the body between the chest and the pelvis that contains the digestive and reproductive (or abdominal) organs, often referred to as the belly.

Abortion The termination of a pregnancy before term; this can be medically induced or spontaneous (known as miscarriage).

Adenoma A non-cancerous cyst or tumour resembling glandular tissue arising from the layer of cells inside organs (epithelium).

Adenomyosis A condition in which the cells that normally line the uterine walls (endometrium) develop in the muscular wall of the uterus tissue, but continue to thicken and shed as part of the menstrual cycle. Unlike endometriosis, these cells are always inside the uterus.

Amniotic fluid The clear, watery fluid that surrounds a foetus in the uterus, cushioning it as the mother moves around and allowing the foetus to move freely.

Amniotic sac The membranous 'bag' surrounding a foetus in the uterus, which is filled with amniotic fluid.

Anaemia A condition in which the concentration of the oxygen-carrying pigment (haemoglobin) in red blood cells is too low. It can result because there are insufficient red blood cells or because those that are circulating are defective. It is not a disease, but a feature of different disorders.

Anaesthetic Literally means loss of sensation. In medicine, anaesthetics are used to numb sensation in certain areas (local anaesthetic), or to induce sleep, for example for surgery (general anaesthetic).

Anal sex A form of sex in which a man's penis enters the anal passage of his partner.

Androgen Hormone that promotes the development and maintenance of male characteristics.

Antenatal Literally the time before birth of a baby. The term is mostly used to describe the care a mother receives during pregnancy prior to the birth.

Antibiotic drugs A group of drugs used to treat bacterial infections. They are sometimes offered to prevent infection if the immune system is impaired.

GLOSSARY OF WOMEN'S HEALTH

Bacteria (single = bacterium) Single-celled organisms abundant in air, soil and water, that are mostly harmless to humans. Some, such as gut bacteria, are beneficial and help break down food. A few, so-called pathogens, can cause disease.

Barrier method of contraception Forms of birth control, such as a condom or cap, that physically prevent a sperm reaching an egg.

Benign A growth or tumour that is not cancerous. It may continue to grow in situ, but it will not spread to other parts of the body.

Bilateral salpingo-oophorectomy Surgical procedure in which the ovaries and fallopian tubes are removed, often carried out as keyhole surgery.

Bi-manual examination A form of examination used to check internal organs in which the practitioner places one hand on the lower part of the person's abdomen and at the same time inserts two fingers into their vagina.

Biopsy A diagnostic test in which a small amount of tissue or a few cells are removed from the body for microscopic examination.

Birth control Any means of controlling fertility to prevent pregnancy, commonly described as contraception.

Bloating A feeling of fullness or swelling in the abdomen, possibly as a result of gas in the intestines, overeating, food intolerances or constipation.

Blood clot A mass of blood that forms if blood platelets, proteins and cells stick together. It can be carried around the body in the bloodstream or can become attached to the wall of a blood vessel (thrombus).

Body mass index (BMI) A means of assessing whether a person is a healthy weight by measuring both weight and height – weight in kg/lbs is divided by height in metres/inches squared – then plotting the calculation on a chart, which gives a number, for example anything between 18.5–24.9 is a healthy weight, above 25 is overweight and above 30 is obese.

Caesarean section/delivery Also called a C-section, this is an operation to deliver a baby through an incision in the abdomen. It is usually performed if a vaginal delivery is medically risky or because a birth becomes difficult (emergency Caesarean).

Cardiovascular disease Disorders and diseases that affect the heart and blood vessels.

Cervical mucus The slippery discharge secreted by the cervix that makes it easier for sperm to swim up the vagina; its consistency changes during the menstrual cycle.

GLOSSARY OF WOMEN'S HEALTH

Cervical screening A regular screening test offered every 3–5 years in women aged 25–65 that assesses the health of the cervix. Cells are taken from the cervix to check for types of human papillomavirus (HPV) that can cause cancerous changes.

Cervix The opening in the lower end of the uterus that leads to the vagina.

Chaperone A person who accompanies another, for example to a medical appointment.

Cisgender (cis) A person whose gender identity is the same as that identified at birth.

Clitoris Part of the female genitalia, this is a small sensitive erectile organ located just below the pubic bone, partly enclosed by the labia.

Clot *see* blood clot

Coeliac disease A condition in which the small intestine is hypersensitive to gluten, the protein found in wheat, rye and barley. Eating gluten causes the immune system to attack and damage the gut tissues, and as a result the person cannot absorb nutrients.

Cognitive function Term used to describe mental processes involved with the acquisition of knowledge, information processing and reasoning.

Coil A small T-shaped device inserted in the uterus to prevent pregnancy. There are two types: a copper coil (intra-uterine device or IUD) and a hormone-releasing coil (intra-uterine system or IUS).

Combined oral contraceptive pill Contraception in the form of a pill that contains artificial versions of the naturally occurring hormones progesterone and oestrogen.

Conception The beginning of pregnancy marked by the fertilization of an egg (ovum) by a sperm.

Condom A sheath-shaped barrier device used to prevent pregnancy and prevent sexually transmitted infections. Condoms can be placed over the penis, or female versions (femidoms) are inserted into the vagina.

Contraception A means of controlling fertility to prevent pregnancy with barrier methods, coils or hormones.

Contraceptive injection An injection that releases the hormone progesterone into the bloodstream for longer-term pregnancy prevention; the effects can last between 8 and 13 weeks depending on the type.

Contraceptive implant Long-term form of contraception in which a small, flexible plastic rod is placed under the skin.

Contractions, uterine Rhythmic spasms of the muscles in the walls of the uterus that occur during childbirth.

Copper coil A small T-shaped implement inserted into the uterus as a form of contraception. This can be fitted at any point in the menstrual cycle.

Corpus luteum A cyst, or cluster of cells, which develops in the ovary during every menstrual cycle, just after an egg (ovum) leaves the ovary.

Crabs *see* Pubic lice

Cramps, period Known as dysmenorrhoea, cramps are painful sensations that can occur when the body releases the hormone-like substances called prostaglandins that cause the uterus to contract to expel its lining before and during a menstrual period.

Cyclical HRT A form of hormone replacement therapy (HRT) offered to women who have menopausal symptoms but who also still have their periods.

Depression A mood disorder that results in persistent feelings of sadness and hopelessness. Symptoms vary depending on the severity.

Diabetes A long-term metabolic disease characterized by high levels of blood sugar (glucose) in the body. Blood sugar is usually broken down by the hormone insulin. Diabetes can develop because the body produces no insulin (Type 1) or because the body cannot use the insulin it produces (Type 2) – the latter is often reversible.

Gestational diabetes A form of diabetes that can develop in pregnancy; this often resolves after pregnancy.

Diagnosis The process of identifying the nature of an illness by examination and assessment of the symptoms.

Diaphragm A barrier method of contraception that is fitted into the vagina to cover the cervix before vaginal sex.

Discharge Fluid that comes out of the body.

Early menopause This is the onset of menopause before the age of 40, and is also known as premature menopause or premature ovarian insufficiency (POI).

Egg A mature female reproductive cell (ovum) released from an ovary that, if fertilized, can develop into an embryo.

Ejaculation The action of ejecting semen from a male's body.

Embryo Human offspring in the process of development from fertilized egg to a foetus.

Emergency contraception This is contraception that can be given after unprotected sex to prevent a pregnancy. There are two forms: a person can take the morning-after pill, or a coil can be inserted.

Endometriosis A condition that occurs when microscopic cells similar to those found in the lining of the uterus – known as the endometrium – are distributed outside the uterus.

Endometrium The inner lining of the uterus.

Episiotomy A surgical cut that can be made at the entrance of the vagina to help a difficult birth and prevent perineum tearing.

Fallopian tube One of two tubes that extend from the top of the uterus towards the ovaries, in which fertilization takes place. The ovum moves along the tube towards the main body of the uterus and the sperm travels from the uterus towards the tube.

Family planning, *see* Contraception

Fasting cholesterol test A blood test to check for cholesterol levels, for which the person is normally asked not to eat for 12 hours beforehand.

Fertility A person or couple's ability to produce offspring, which is dependent on age and health.

Fertilization The point at which a sperm enters an egg (ovum).

Fibroid A benign, slow-growing tumour formed of smooth muscle and connective tissue that can develop in the uterus. There can be one or more and the size can vary.

Follicle A small cavity in the body, for example a hair follicle. In an ovary, follicles are small sac-like, fluid-filled pouches, each of which contains one ovum (egg).

GP A general practitioner, or family doctor, is a doctor who assesses and treats common medical conditions, and refers patients to other medical disciplines for more specialist treatment when necessary.

Gender The sex that a person identifies themselves as, such as male, female or non-binary.

Gender affirmation therapy Any of several therapies, psychological and physical, that are offered to a person to help them live in their preferred gender identity.

Gender diverse A place that accommodates people of different genders; also an umbrella term used to address the spectrum of different gender identities.

Genitals A person's external sex organs.

GLOSSARY OF WOMEN'S HEALTH

Gestation The period of time between conception and birth during which an infant develops in the uterus, normally 40 weeks or 9 months.

Gynaecological cancer A cancer that affects any part of the reproductive system of a female.

Gynaecologist Doctor or surgeon specializing in the branch of medicine that focuses on female health and the female reproductive system.

Hormone Chemical messengers released into the bloodstream by certain organs that have a specific effect on tissues somewhere else in the body.

Hot flush A common symptom of the menopause, caused by hormonal imbalances, in which a person experiences a sudden rise in body temperature especially in the upper body, often accompanied by sweating, and looks flushed.

Hyperthyroidism Also known as overactive thyroid, a condition that results in overproduction of thyroid hormones. Symptoms include increase in heart rate, appetite and sweating, as well as weight loss.

Hypothyroidism Also known as underactive thyroid, a condition that results in inadequate levels of thyroid hormones, causing tiredness, lethargy and weight gain.

Hysterectomy The surgical removal of the uterus. The most common type involves only the uterus and cervix; sometimes the ovaries and fallopian tubes are also removed.

Implantation The point at which a fertilized egg (ovum) attaches itself to the wall of the uterus – this normally happens six days after fertilization.

Incontinence The involuntary passing of urine, which can be caused by injury, weakness or disease of the urinary tract.

Infertility Inability to produce a baby. This can be a result of a problem in the male or female reproductive systems, or both.

Inflammation Pain, swelling, heat and redness in one or several areas of the body as a result of an injury or infection.

Insomnia The inability to fall asleep or to stay asleep for any length of time. Causes can be physical, psychological or environmental.

Insulin The hormone produced by the pancreas that controls blood sugar levels in the body.

Insulin resistance A condition in which the body's cells do not respond properly to insulin whether it's produced by the body, or injected (in those with diabetes).

GLOSSARY OF WOMEN'S HEALTH

Intercourse Also known as sexual intercourse, this is physical contact between two individuals that involves genitalia of at least one of them.

Intra-uterine device (IUD) Small 'T'-shaped, non-hormonal device (coil) that is inserted into the uterus as a form of contraception.

Intra-uterine system (IUS) Small 'T'-shaped, hormone-releasing device (coil) that is inserted into the uterus as a form of contraception.

Keloid scars A scar that continues growing after a wound is healed and can grow to bigger than the original wound.

LGBTQ+ Acronym used to refer to the group of people who identify as lesbian, gay, bisexual, transgender, queer or questioning. The '+' acknowledges that there are other sexual identities, such as intersex and asexual.

Labia majora The outer lips of the female external genitals.

Labia minora The inner lips of the female external genitals.

Labour The process by which an infant is born.

Laparoscopy A surgical procedure in which the interior of the abdomen is examined using a device called a laparoscope, which is inserted through a small hole ('key' hole) made in the abdominal wall.

Libido Level of sexual desire.

Lubricant An oily or slippery substance that can for example be used to reduce friction during intercourse.

MRI scan Short for magnetic resonance imaging, this is a diagnostic technique that produces cross-sectional or three-dimensional images of organs or body structures.

Mammogram A type of X-ray used specifically to examine the breasts for signs of cancer, offered as a form of screening.

Mastectomy Surgical removal of one or both breasts, usually to treat breast cancer.

Menopause The point in a woman's life when menstruation has ceased for 12 months, regardless of other symptoms.

Menstruation The periodic shedding of the lining of a woman's uterus that occurs if they are not pregnant.

Midwife A person trained to assist women in childbirth.

Migraine A type of headache characterized by recurrent attacks of severe pain, usually on one side of the head, which can cause a throbbing sensation.

Mini-pill Also known as the progesterone-only pill (POP), this is a contraceptive pill that contains only progesterone, which works by thickening the cervical mucus and preventing the sperm reaching the egg.

GLOSSARY OF WOMEN'S HEALTH

Miscarriage The loss of a foetus before week 24 of pregnancy.

Morning-after pill, *see* Emergency contraception

Multidisciplinary team Healthcare team that is comprised of a number of different specialties, who work together to assist with a person's medical care.

Myometrium The muscle tissue in the wall of the uterus.

Nausea Feeling sick or the need to vomit.

Needlestick injury Accidental puncture of the skin by a potentially contaminated hypodermic needle, which carries a risk of disease.

Neuropathic or neuropathy Disease or inflammation affecting the peripheral nerves, the nerves that connect to the central nervous system (brain and spinal cord).

NHS The UK's health system – the National Health Service – which includes all healthcare practitioners.

Non-binary A person who does not identify themselves as either male or female.

Obesity A state of being very overweight; a person with a BMI above 30 is described as obese.

Obstetrician A doctor or surgeon specializing in the branch of medicine concerned with childbirth.

Oestrogen(s) A group of hormones essential for the maintenance of female characteristics of the body.

Oestrogen-receptor-positive breast cancer (ER+) A type of breast cancer with cells that have receptors that allow them to use oestrogen hormones to grow – so a person can be given medication to reduce the hormone production as a form of treatment.

Off licence Use of a drug or other preparation in a way that is not typically recommended by the manufacturer, but that is still safe.

Oophorectomy Surgical procedure in which the ovaries are removed.

Oral medication Medicines or tablets that are taken by mouth.

Oral sex Sexual activity in which one person's genitals are stimulated by the mouth of another person.

Osteoporosis Loss of bone tissue that causes bones to become brittle/fragile so are more likely to fracture. This is a natural part of ageing, but women lose bone tissue faster after the menopause.

Ovarian cyst Abnormal, fluid-filled swelling that can develop on an ovary.

Ovary One of two glands, positioned either side of the uterus, in which eggs (ova) form and the female hormones oestrogen and progesterone are made.

Ovulation The process of the ovary releasing an egg (ovum).

GLOSSARY OF WOMEN'S HEALTH

Ovum (plural = ova) The mature female reproductive cell released from an ovary that, if fertilized, can develop into an embryo.

Patch An adhesive-plaster-like device that releases medication, for example for HRT or contraception, into the body through the skin; the patch is normally changed every 2–3 weeks.

Pelvis Large bony, basin-like frame at the base of the spine that surrounds and protects the reproductive organs.

Penetration Physical contact between two individuals in which a man puts his penis into the vagina or anus of their partner.

Penis The largest external male sex organ.

Perimenopause The time before the menopause when a woman has symptoms of the menopause, but is still menstruating; this can last up to a decade.

Perinatal phase The weeks immediately before and after the birth of a baby.

Perineum The part of the body between the entrance to the vagina (or the scrotum) and the anus.

Period Also known as menstruation, this is the periodic shedding of the lining of a woman's uterus that occurs if they are not pregnant.

Pessary Medical device placed into the vagina, to correct the position of the uterus or to deliver medication or contraception.

Physiotherapist Healthcare professional who provides physical therapy treatment to help prevent or reduce joint stiffness and aid movement.

Pituitary gland Situated under the brain, this is the most important gland of the endocrine (hormone-producing) system. Called the master gland, it controls and regulates all the other endocrine glands and many body processes.

Placenta The organ formed in the uterus during pregnancy that supports and nourishes the foetus.

Placental abruption Separation of the placenta from the wall of the uterus during pregnancy or labour before the baby is born; this is life-threatening to mother and baby.

Polyp A growth, often from a stalk, that projects from the wall of an organ, such as the cervix, uterus, or nose. Some are cancerous and need to be removed.

Polycystic ovary syndrome (PCOS) A condition that can cause cysts on the ovaries. Confusingly the syndrome can also cause other effects (such as excess hair, weight gain, oily skin, or irregular or absent periods) without the presence of cysts on the ovaries.

GLOSSARY OF WOMEN'S HEALTH

Post-menopause The life stage of a woman, or person assigned a woman at birth, after the menopause.

Post-natal The first weeks after the birth of a baby.

Post-partum The hours immediately after the birth of a baby.

Premature menopause Menopause that begins when a woman is under the age of 40 years.

Progesterone Hormone made in the ovaries that is essential to the functioning of the female reproductive system.

Progesterone-only pill (POP) *see* Mini pill

Progestogen drugs A group of drugs containing properties similar to naturally occurring hormone progesterone that are used in contraceptives.

Prolapse Displacement of an organ, for example the uterus, from its normal place in the body.

Puberty The time during which a girl (or boy) becomes sexually mature.

Pubic lice Tiny parasitic insects, often called crabs, that can attach themselves to the skin and hair of the areas around the genitals. Spread by close physical contact they cause intense itching; lice and/or eggs may be visible.

Pulmonary embolism Obstruction of one of the arterial blood vessels in the lungs by a blood clot. Clots can form in the lungs or be carried there from another part of the circulatory system by the blood.

Screening The regular testing of apparently healthy members of the population to check for signs of diseases.

Semen The sperm-containing fluid released from the penis during ejaculation/orgasm.

Sequential HRT A form of hormone replacement therapy for women who still menstruate that involves taking one hormone daily (oestrogen), then additional progesterone for part (normally half) of the month.

Sexuality A person's identity in relation to the genders they are attracted to, and/or how they identify their own sexuality. It also describes a person's attitude and behaviour towards sex and physical intimacy with others.

Sexually transmitted diseases (STDs) Diseases that are transmitted through sexual contact with another person.

Side effect The secondary response caused by a drug beyond the intended therapeutic effects.

Smear test Routine screening test offered every 3–5 years to all women (or those assigned female at birth) aged 25–65 in which cells are collected

GLOSSARY OF WOMEN'S HEALTH

from the cervix to check for types of human papillomavirus (HPV) that can cause cancerous changes in the cervix.

Speculum Device placed in the vagina by a healthcare professional so that the cervix can be checked, and a smear test can be carried out.

Sperm The male sex cell that is responsible for fertilization of an egg (ovum).

Spotting Light traces of blood that can indicate the end of a period, or that are sometimes seen around ovulation.

Stress incontinence Involuntary loss of urine that occurs, for example, when a person coughs or lifts a heavy object, because the muscles at the exit to the urinary tract (sphincter) are weakened, for example after childbirth.

Surrogacy The process of carrying and giving birth to a baby for another person. The birth mother then hands over custody of the baby to that person.

Swab Small absorbent pad or cloth (generally sterile) used in surgery or by a healthcare professional to clean a wound, apply medication or take a specimen.

Synthetic A chemically made substance that imitates a naturally occurring product.

Systemic Medical treatment using substances/drugs that travel throughout the body.

Testosterone The hormone that stimulates the development of, and maintains, secondary male characteristics.

Tinnitus Continuous or intermittent ringing, buzzing or roaring sound in one, or more commonly both, ears.

Topical A medication or treatment applied directly to an area (of skin, for example).

Toxic shock syndrome A rare, but potentially life-threatening, condition caused by harmful bacteria getting into the body and releasing toxins. It is sometimes associated with tampon use in young women.

Trans man Person living as a man who was assigned female gender at birth.

Trans woman Person living as a woman who was assigned male gender at birth.

Transdermal Application of a drug through the skin, typically via an adhesive patch.

Transgender, or trans A person who is not living as the gender they were assigned at birth.

Transvaginal ultrasound scan An ultrasound scan carried out using a probe inserted into the vagina, *see also* Ultrasound scan

GLOSSARY OF WOMEN'S HEALTH

Trimester One of the three 'periods' of pregnancy, each covering around one-third of the pregnancy.

Triple-negative cancer An aggressive, fast-growing form of breast cancer in which the cells do not have hormone receptors that they need for growth.

Ultrasound scan A diagnostic tool that involves passing high-frequency sound waves through the body – the reflected echoes build a picture of the organs, or foetus for example, visible on a screen.

Unprotected sex Sexual intercourse with no form of contraception.

Urethra The opening, or sphincter, at the end of the ureter through which urine flows out of the body.

Urge incontinence The uncontrolled leakage of urine that occurs when a person feels a sudden urge to pee and is unable to stop the flow.

Uterine fibroids (leiomyomas) Noncancerous growths of the uterus.

Uterus Largest internal female reproductive organ in which a foetus remains during pregnancy.

Vaccine A medical preparation that is given to induce immunity to an infectious disease. Some require several doses to take effect and for others one dose provides life immunity.

Vagina The muscular tube, or canal, between the external female genitalia (vulva) and the internal organs of the cervix and the uterus.

Vaginal mucus Slimy substance secreted by the vagina that varies in consistency.

Vaginal atrophy Thinning of the vaginal walls, which can cause dryness and irritation.

Vaginal oestrogen A form of oestrogen (female hormone) that is administered in the form of a pessary or cream into the vagina.

Virus Simple, small microorganisms that replicate inside cells and can cause disease.

Vulva The external female genitals.

Vulvodynia Pain and discomfort in and around the vulval, vaginal and groin area. Can be generalised or provoked.

Withdrawal method A method to avoid pregnancy when the penis is removed from the vagina before orgasm/ejaculation to prevent sperm entering the vagina.

Womb The non-medical word used to describe the uterus.

X-ray A diagnostic tool that involves passing electromagnetic radiation of short wavelength and high energy through the body to view bones, organs and internal tissues.

RESOURCES

FAIR HEALTHCARE ACCESS FOR ALL
Women's health & disability
Sisters of Frida organization, a collective of disabled women: www.sisofrida.org

Trans patient training for doctors
GPs can access an excellent module on the Royal College of GP's LGBT Health Hub: www.elearning.rcgp.org.uk
The Gender GP online clinic also contains a wealth of useful information for physicians and patients: www.gendergp.com

INFORMATION AND HELP DURING PUBERTY YEARS
Periods
Wellbeing of Women charity: www.wellbeingofwomen.org.uk

Period tracking apps
Flo: www.flo.health
Clue: www.helloclue.com
Ovia Health: www.oviahealth.com

Period inequality
Plan International: www.plan-international.org
The Trussell Trust: www.trusselltrust.org
Binti International: www.bintiperiod.org

Premenstrual dysphoric disorder
International Association for Premenstrual Disorders (IAPMD) self-screening test: www.iapmd.org/self-screen

Violence against women & girls
Childline: www.childline.org.uk; Helpline: 0800 1111
Women's Aid: www.womensaid.org.uk
SWGfL, a charity offering support for online abuse: www.swgfl.org.uk
Karma Nirvana, working to end honour-based abuse: www.karmanirvana.org.uk

RESOURCES

Female genital mutilation
FGM-related help, advice and support is available from a number of charitable organizations.
FGM National Women's Group: www.fgmnationalgroup.org/
Action Aid: www.actionaid.org.uk
Oxfam: www.oxfam.org
UN Women: www.unwomen.org
Women & Girls Network: www.wgn.org.uk

Contraception & sexual health
Brook, offering confidential advice for young people: www.brook.org.uk
Health for Teens: www.healthforteens.co.uk
NHS advice and information: www.letstalkaboutit.nhs.uk

Unplanned pregnancies & ending a pregnancy
Brook, offering confidential advice for young people: www.brook.org.uk
British Pregnancy Advisory Service: www.bpas.org.uk
Pregnancy Crisis Helpline:
  www.pregnancycrisishelpline.org.uk;
  Helpline: 0800 368 9296
National Unplanned Pregnancy Advice Service:
  www.nupas.co.uk
Marie Stopes Clinics for abortion care services:
  www.msichoices.org.uk
Planned Parenthood, a US-based organization for advice and guidance: www.plannedparenthood.org

Sexually transmitted diseases
The following websites contain some really useful information:
Brook, offering confidential advice for young people: www.brook.org.uk
Better2Know, offering sexual health testing services: www.better2know.co.uk
Terrence Higgins Trust, an HIV and sexual health charity: www.tht.org.uk

Gender identity
The following resources contain some useful information:
Gender Identity Development Service: www.gids.nhs.uk
Trans Actual: www.transactual.org.uk
Welsh Gender Service: www.cavuhb.nhs.wales/our-services/welsh-gender-service

RESOURCES

National Gender Identity Clinical Network for Scotland: www.ngicns.scot.nhs.uk/gender-identity-clinics

Regional Gender Identity Service for Northern Ireland: www.belfasttrust.hscni.net/service/regional-gender-identity-service/

Regional Gender Identity Clinic for Northern Ireland (under-18s): www.familysupportni.gov.uk/Search/Details/5033?slug=gender-identity-clinic--camhs-belfast

Egg preservation for trans people

Human Fertilisation & Embryology Authority (HFEA): www.hfea.gov.uk

Mental health & trans people

Stonewall, a UK-based charity that stands for the freedom, equity and potential of all lesbian, gay, bi, trans, queer, questioning and ace (LGBTQ+) people: www.stonewall.org.uk

Young people visiting a GP alone

NSPCC, offering advice about the Gillick competence and Fraser guidelines: https://learning.nspcc.org.uk/child-protection-system/gillick-competence-fraser-guidelines

STATISTICS RESOURCES

Page 42: 8.9% of the residents of England and Wales did not have English as their main language in 2021 (Office for National Statistics 2021 Census, 29 November 2022. www.ons.gov.uk/peoplepopulationandcommunity/culturalidentity/language/bulletins/languageenglandandwales/census2021)

Page 67: 13% of UK schoolgirls missed a day of school every month due to their period ('Nearly two million girls miss school because of their period', Plan International website, 20 October 2021. www.plan-uk.org/media-centre/nearly-two-million-girls-in-the-uk-miss-school-because-of-their-period#:~:text=Nearly%20two%20million%20girls%20(64,children's%20charity%20Plan%20International%20UK)

Page 87: A year's worth of disposable period products contributes 5.3kg of C02 ('Which Period Products are Best for the Environment?', by Leah Rodriguez, Global Citizen website, 27 May 2021. www.globalcitizen.org/en/content/best-period-products-for-the-environment/)

Page 92: The average woman in the UK will spend up to £18,450 on products geared towards her period over a lifetime ('Women Spend More than

RESOURCES

£18,000 on Having Periods in Their Lifetime, Study Reveals', by Rachel Moss, The Huffington Post UK website, 3 September 2015. www.huffingtonpost.co.uk/2015/09/03/women-spend-thousands-on-periods-tampon-tax_n_8082526.html)

Page 93: A 2017 survey revealed that nearly half of daughters in the UK said they'd feel uncomfortable discussing periods with their fathers ('1 in 4 UK women don't understand their menstrual cycle', Action Aid website, 23 May 2017. https://www.actionaid.org.uk/blog/news/2017/05/24/1-in-4-uk-women-dont-understand-their-menstrual-cycle)

Page 114: Globally 29% of all women of reproductive age are affected by anaemia (The Global Prevalence of Anaemia in 2011 by World Health Organization, 2015. apps.who.int/iris/bitstream/handle/10665/177094/9789241564960_eng.pdf)

Page 133: 27% of couples practising the withdrawal method will get pregnant each year ('Withdrawal as pregnancy prevention and associated risk factors among US high school students: findings from the 2011 National Youth Risk Behavior Survey' by Nicole Liddon, Emily O'Malley Olsen, Marion Carter and Kendra Hatfield-Timajchy, Contraception: An international reproductive health journal, February 2016. www.contraceptionjournal.org/article/S0010-7824(15)00571-5/fulltext)

Page 172: 46% of trans people in the UK have experienced suicidal thoughts (LGBT in Britain Health Report, by Chaka L Bachmann (Stonewall) and Becca Gooch (YouGov), 7 November 2018. https://www.stonewall.org.uk/resources/lgbt-britain-health-2018

INDEX

abortion 158–9
acne 64, 136
Action Aid 91
acupuncture 106, 108
adrenalin 74
AIDS (acquired immunodeficiency syndrome) 166
alcohol 106, 108
alveoli 16, 17
anaemia 113–14, 136
anatomy, female 9–36, 61
antidepressants 108, 110
anus 12, 13, 14, 15, 125, 127
Asian ethnic minorities 39, 41, 42

bacterial infections 119, 122, 123, 125
bacterial vaginosis 122, 123, 125–6
Bat Mitzvah 97
beauty products 120–1
Binti International 90, 100
Black ethnic minorities 39
bladder 12, 13, 127
body shape 63
boys, educating on women's health 62
bras 25–9, 63
breasts 16–29, 170
  anatomy of 16–17
  bras 25–9, 63
  breast cancer 19
  changes during puberty 63, 67
  self examination 9, 19–23, 39–40

cancer
  breast cancer 19
  cancer screening 51
  gynaecological cancers 31, 116, 136, 153, 165
carers, advice for 61–2, 91–3
cervix 10, 11, 13, 66
  cervical cancer 165
  infections 122, 123
chaperones 40, 41
chest binding 172
chlamydia 162, 163–4
clitoris 13, 14, 15, 31, 34
cognitive impairment 46–7
combined contraceptive pill 110, 112, 135–6, 145, 161, 169
condoms 148–51
contraception 112–13, 131–56, 168
  barrier methods 148–53, 161
  hormonal contraception 133–46, 169
  withdrawal method & emergency contraception 134, 154–6
corpus luteum 67
cortisol 74
crabs 165
cravings 111–12
cultural attitudes 97–101
cystitis 127, 128

diaphragm 151–3
disability 45–7, 49
discharge 33, 64, 66, 67, 74, 119, 125
  colours of 121–3

INDEX

discrimination 37, 48, 49, 54, 89, 99, 167
dysmenorrhoea 103

eating disorders 170
eggs (ovum) 10, 11, 66, 67, 70, 111, 135, 145
emergency contraception 134, 155–6
emotions 63
endometriosis 73, 112, 116, 138, 168
endometrium 11, 67, 70–1
  contraception and 141, 143
  periods and 10, 66, 75, 103
environment, period products and 86–7
ethnic minorities 39–43, 89, 174

fallopian tubes 10, 11, 13, 66
female genital mutilation (FMG) 118
fertility, trans individuals 169–70
fibroids 73, 112, 116
follicle stimulating hormone (FSH) 65–6
follicles 66, 67, 70
follicular phase 66, 70, 71
food cravings 111–12
free bleeding 83
fungal infections 119, 125

gender dysphoria 86, 168, 170
gender dysphoria clinics (GDC) 52, 171
gender identity 52, 171
Gender Identity Development Service (GIDS) 171
Gill, Manjit 90, 100
gonadotropin-releasing hormone analogues (GnR Ha) 110
gonorrhoea 162, 164

gynaecological cancers 31, 116, 136, 153, 165

hair 63, 98–9
headaches 93–4
healthcare access for all 37–55
height 63
herpes virus 163
Hinduism 97
HIV (human immunodeficiency virus) 162, 166
hormones 65–6, 106–7
  hormonal contraception 133–46
  see also individual hormones
human papillomavirus (HPV) 132, 165
hygiene, genital 119–21

implants, contraceptive 108, 112, 139–40, 169
injections, contraceptive 108, 112, 140–2
International Association for Premenstrual Disorders (IAPMD) 109, 110, 111
interpreters 40, 41, 46
Islam 42, 97, 99
IUD (intra-uterine device) coil 146–8, 155–6
IUS (intra-uterine system) coil 113, 142–4, 169

Judaism 99

Kamaruddin, Dr Kamilla 53

labia 13, 14, 15, 31, 35
language barriers 40, 41, 42
lice, pubic 165
lobules 16, 17

INDEX

long-acting reversible contraceptives (LARCS) 108
luteal phase 67, 70, 71, 111
luteinizing hormone (LH) 65–6

magnesium glycinate 105
medical appointments 40
menorrhagia 112
menstrual cycle 10
   health & comfort issues during 103–16
Menstrual Hygiene Day 91
menstruation *see* periods
mental health, trans individuals 170
milk ducts 16, 17
mini-pill 112, 137–8, 169
Mirena™ IUS coil 143
morning after pill 155, 156
myths 97–100

nipples 16, 17
non-binary people 86, 167–72
NuvaRing™ 144–6

oestrogen 65–6
   contraception 135, 145
   effect on breasts 19, 51
   fluctuations in levels 12, 19, 67, 74, 109
oral sex 132
ovaries 10, 11, 13, 66, 67, 70, 111, 135, 145
ovulation phase 66, 67, 70, 71, 74, 142

pads 79–81, 87
pain
   pain relief 105–6, 127–8, 143, 147
   period pain 103–6
parents, advice for 61–2, 91–3

Pausitivity 42, 43
pectoral muscles 16, 17
perineum 12, 13, 14, 15, 35
period cups 85, 86
period pants 82, 86
periods 10, 64, 65–106
   and anaemia 113–14, 136
   changes to your flow 75
   colour & consistency 74, 75
   cultural attitudes towards 97–101
   heavy periods 112–13, 114, 115, 135, 136, 137
   length of 72
   myths and superstitions 97–100
   period inequality 89–90
   period pain 103–6
   period products 78–87, 89, 92
   phases of 65–7, 71
   regularity of 73–4, 136, 170
   starting your 67–8, 92–3, 97
   talking about 91–5
   tracking 75–7
   trans individuals 169
   when to see the doctor 115–16
the Pill 135–6, 145, 161, 169
polycystic ovary syndrome (PCOS) 73, 112, 116, 168
pregnancy, unplanned 157–9
premenstrual dysphoric disorder (PMDD) 109–11, 115, 143
premenstrual syndrome (PMS) 106–9, 168
   symptoms 67, 94, 107, 111, 115
   treating with contraception 138, 143, 145
premenstrual tension (PMT) 107–8
progesterone 65–6, 67, 109
   contraception 135, 137–8, 141–5, 169
prostaglandin 103–4

INDEX

puberty 57–116
pubic area 14, 31–5
pubic lice 165
pyelonephritis 127

Quinceañera 97

reproductive system
   anatomy of 10–15, 11, 13
   self examination 30–5

serotonin 111
sexual abuse 117
sexual health 131–3, 161–6
shame 39, 65, 91, 94, 99
Sisters of Frida 45
skin 64
smear tests 51, 165
smoking 106, 108
South Asian communities 41, 42–3
sport, period products and 87
STDs (sexually transmitted diseases) 122, 123, 131, 148, 149, 150, 161–6
sterilization, female 153
stigma 39, 65, 91, 94, 174
Stonewall 49, 170
stress 73, 74
superstitions 97–100
sweat 63–4
syphilis 164

tampons 84, 87, 98
terminations 158–9
thrush 125, 126
trans individuals 167–72
   bridging prescriptions 53
   changing name & gender details 50
   chest binding 172
   complaints procedure 54
   eating disorders 170
   fertility 169–70
   gender identity 52, 171
   mental health 170
   periods 86, 169
   rights for 49–55
   routine cancer screening 51
   shared care agreements 52–3
   surgery trans policy 50–1
TransActual 49
transcutaneous electrical nerve stimulation (TENS) 106
trichomoniasis 164

underwear, period 82, 86
urethra 12, 13, 14, 15
uterus 10, 11, 13, 64, 66, 70, 103
UTIs (urinary tract infections) 119, 120, 125, 127–9

vagina 12
   anatomy of 10, 11, 13, 14, 15
   caring for your 119–21
   discharge 33, 64, 66, 67, 74, 119, 121–3, 125
   self examination 31, 35
vaginal ring 144–6
violence, against women and girls 117–18
vitamin B1 (thiamine) 105
vulva 10, 12, 14, 30–5, 119–21

withdrawal method 133, 134, 154–5

yeast infections 119, 121, 122–3, 125, 126

ACKNOWLEDGEMENTS

This book and my medical career so far would not have been possible without the help and support of so many people. It's true that it really does take a village! And in particular I'd like to thank the following people and organizations.

I want to say a huge thank you to my family. My parents, whose duas (prayers) and guidance continue to support me, and my siblings, Irfan, Imran, Saba and Ali, who will always be my best friends. My husband, Khalid, is a pillar of support, a dad to our three boys, and a soundboard for the choices I make. To my children, Haris, Qasim and Adam, who are my world and provide so much fun in my life. To the Pakistani women in my community: when I first arrived in the UK, they provided so much food, love, education and embraced us with open arms. These incredible women continue to teach me the facets of womanhood to this day.

When it comes to medicine and women's health, I am fully aware that I stand on the shoulders of giants, in particular Dr Louise Newson, who gave me the courage to push my understanding on HRT and menopause care and translate that to my South Asian community. Dr Annice Mukherjee made me understand the impact of hormones in women, and to Dr Radikha Vohra, Dr Aziza Sesey, Dr Liz O'Riordan, Dr Philippa Kaye, Dr Zoe Williams, Dr Larissa, Dr Sara Hyat, Dr Punam Krishan, Dr Naomi Potter – whose book with Davina McCall I contributed to – thank you for

ACKNOWLEDGEMENTS

your support. Thank you also to my colleagues from the US from whom I learn so much: Dr Karen Tang, Dr Mary Claire Haver and Dr Rachel Rubin.

To all the people who have contributed towards getting this book into its current state, thank you. In particular, Dr Ajay Verma who has been immensely helpful in providing me with education and support when proofreading sections of the book, and Dr Kamilah Kamaruddin, who is a voice for trans rights in the medical community and gave her wise insight into the sections on healthcare for trans people.

A huge thank you to my family at Wellbeing of Women, especially Dame Lesley Regan, Janet Lindsay, who brought me on as an ambassador, and my fellow ambassador Rosie Nixon, for her constant support. Thanks also to Manjit Gill MBE from Binti Period, whose campaigning about periods is invaluable and who contributed her knowledge about the myths around menstrual cycles, and to Hibo Wardere and Nimko Ali OBE, whose advice helped me to write about FGM with clarity and authority. I'm eternally grateful for grassroots campaigners who do so much for women's health: Diane Danzebrink, founder of Menopause Support; Elizabeth Carr-Ellis From Pausitivity; and South Asian breast cancer campaigns and campaigners, Sakoon Through Cancer, Iyna Butt, Kreena Dhiman and Bep Dhaliwal. And thank you to the charities: The Eve Appeal, Jo's Cervical Cancer Trust, Breast Cancer Now, Lichen Sclerosus and Vulval Cancer UK Awareness who have been a wealth of information and have always supported my work.

ACKNOWLEDGEMENTS

Thanks to Jan Croxson, my agent, who found me in 2019, met me for 30 seconds and said she'd like to sign me. I was gobsmacked that somebody would take a punt on a hijab-wearing, slightly potty-mouthed, Muslim woman with three kids and take me into the world of media along with Borra Garson and Louise Leftwich. To Davina McCall for being so supportive and lifter of women.

To Kate Muir who originally asked me to be involved with *Davina McCall: Sex, Myths and the Menopause*. To Eleanor Mills who helped me to write about women's health and who brought me on as an ambassador for Noon.

A huge thank you to the BBC and ITV teams. Thanks also to my BBC Three Counties Radio team, especially Louise Parry, and Toby Friedner, who tried to teach me the art of presenting on a Sunday morning when I've had little to no breakfast and half a cup of tea, but with whom it's been an absolute blast to learn – there is more to presenting than I was ever aware of.

Thank you Baroness Sayeeda Warsi, Saira Khan, Anita Rani, Pippa Vosper, Lavina Mehta MBE, Meera Bhogal, Tessy Ojo CBE, for always championing my work. My HerSpirit friends: Mel Berry, Holly Woodford and Professor Greg Whyte, who literally motivate me to do exercise and get fitter, stronger, healthier in every way because I consume more chocolate than I should!

A huge thank you to my NHS surgery, in particular my supportive colleagues Dr Heather White, Dr Kirsten Riemer and Dr Lee Mitchell. To all my colleagues at OSD Healthcare who helped me set up a private women's health

ACKNOWLEDGEMENTS

clinic to my own exacting specifications, even getting Entonox for pain relief in my coil insertion clinics. And to my NHS patients, who through their lived experience, have been more of an education than any medical textbook.

A massive thank you to Stephanie Jackson for believing in the vision of this book and taking on this huge gauntlet of a project. I'm so grateful to Jo Lake and Han, whose wisdom and advice I very much appreciated. I'm also grateful to Pauline Bache, Jaz Bahra, and Liliana Rasmussen for all their help, without Liliana's illustrations, this book would not have the soul that it does have.

My teachers at the Misbourne School, in particular my head teacher David Selman, who refused to make me headgirl so I could concentrate on my A-levels and become the first student from the school to go on to study medicine, thank you. Mrs Carol Taylor who provided me with mentorship and tissues as I cried in her office on a practically daily basis for fear of failure (she always had shortbread biscuits and tea); Ms Lorraine Cummings who helped me do my UCAS application to get into Queen Mary's University of London Barts and the London School of Medicine. And to all the professors, friends, lecturers at Barts who put me on my journey to becoming a doctor.

Finally to nine-year-old me, the little Nighat, who was so lost and had left everything she had known in Pakistan. She was in an alien world, never having the right clothing for the wet and cold weather, not understanding the new food and way of life, but she also gained all these freedoms and was able to not be hindered as a girl. Moving here, I felt

ACKNOWLEDGEMENTS

a bittersweet loss of my life in Pakistan but I also realized a love of what I found in the UK. There's no other place like my hometown of Chesham. When I came here as that young girl I was constantly battling to try and find my identity, so I want to say thank you to that girl, because she persevered with a smile (still, when I'm nervous I smile, which is why I'm always smiling on TV!) and for gradually loosened the shackles of the patriarchy in a small way, being slightly rebellious and finding company in medicine. Because of that, this book is for all the other people who have a sense of loss of identity and loss of grounding – and who every now and then say to themselves, What am I doing? I hope that you can at least feel like you have a handle on and an understanding of your own body and how to best care for it, as a helping hand along the way.

ABOUT THE AUTHOR

Dr Nighat Arif is a GP specializing in women's health and family planning with over 16 years of experience in the NHS and private practice. She is based in Buckinghamshire, UK and is able to consult fluently with patients in Urdu and Punjabi. Dr Nighat is a medical educator and provides teaching to local trainee GPs as well as at national and international conferences. Dr Nighat was nominated for the National Bevan Prize for Health and Wellbeing to acknowledge her exceptional commitment to advancing wellbeing in her community. Dr Nighat has worked to raise awareness on menopause and women's healthcare in Black and Asian women; she presented her clinical work at the 'Menopause in the Workplace' Parliamentary committee hearing. She has also worked with Team Halo, a United Nations (UN) initiative to bring an end to the pandemic and presented at the G7 Global Vaccine Confidence Summit that led to her being awarded an Honorary Doctorate Degree in Science at London City University for Women's Health, Public Health and Inclusion. She is the honorary recipient of the 2023 SHE Award and received a Points of Light Award 2023 from the UK Prime Minister in recognition of her exceptional service to raising awareness for women's health in the UK.

Dr Nighat is the resident doctor on *BBC Breakfast*, ITV'S *This Morning* and BBC *LookEast*, and she hosts her own Sunday Breakfast show on BBC3 Counties

ABOUT THE AUTHOR

Radio. Dr Nighat was also a contributor on the Channel 4 documentary *Davina McCall: Sex, Lies and the Menopause* and has made guest appearances on numerous podcasts tackling taboos around women's health. Dr Nighat has regularly written for various publications including *Stylist, HELLO, Red, Good Housekeeping* and *Women in Medicine* and her work around menopause has featured in *British Vogue*. She is also an ambassador of the global charity Wellbeing of Women, Roald Dahl's Marvellous Children's Charity, The Good Grief Trust, HerSpirit, Sikh Forgiveness and Upon Noon. She lives in Buckinghamshire with her husband and three sons.

@DrNighatArif